Praise for *The Naked Warrior*

"Mr. Tsatsouline ha[s] ... [trainin]g for the 21st century! Recently retired from ... used to agonize over the archaic athletic trainin[g] ... sis; Now, Pavel's research can yield a much more ... ackage."
—John McKean, six ... [Wo]rld Champion

"With *The Naked Warrior*, Pavel has moved the art of exercise without weights to a new level. Now, whether you have weights or not, there is no reason not to get into top shape!"
—Arthur Drechsler, author "*The Weightlifting Encyclopedia*"

"*The Naked Warrior* is the best book I have read on strength building since **Only the Strong Shall Survive**. I really enjoyed it."
—Ed O'Neill, actor

"The tools Pavel explains in *The Naked Warrior* will help my Olympic style weight lifters gain the core strength they need to put additional kg on their totals. Thanks Pavel for such a great work!!"
—Mike Burgener, Sr international weightlifting coach

"For martial artists who don't wish to weight train or just don't have the time *The Naked Warrior* program is **the way** to go to enhance strength. You can practice martial skills without the information offered in *The Naked Warrior*, but you risk not operating at full potential."
—George Demetriou, Modern Warrior Defensive Tactics Institute, NYC

"*The Naked Warrior* has caused me to completely re-evaluate the way I look at calisthenics...it allows us in the field to still train for great strength with only our bodies and that's **like money in the bank!**"
—SSgt. Nate Morrison, USAF, Pararescue Combatives Course Project Manager

"If you are that rare breed who will never settle for anything less than the best you can possibly be, *The Naked Warrior* is the book for you. It teaches people of all levels of fitness how to reach levels that they might never have thought possible. **I improved my deadlift from 465 to 505 in one month.** My "pistol" is now rock bottom, and a Gold's gym musclehead called me a *Cirque de Soleil performer.*"
—Randy Part, Santa Monica, CA

"*The Naked Warrior* is pure gold. If you follow Pavel's advice as laid out in this book, you will get stronger, regardless of your current level of strength. And you'll do it safely - and quicker than you thought possible, with less effort than you thought imaginable. **Pavel's works have changed my life**, and made training at the age of 44 more fun and effective than ever."
—John Quigley, Camp Hill, PA

"No words can accurately convey the depth of my appreciation for Pavel and the light he has cast on Russian strength and health systems. He's deepened and broadened the path between world-class performance and the average individual who wants to increase strength and fitness. **This information is worth its weight in gold.**"
—Steven Barnes, North West

"I practiced yoga for years and train hard to be a strong rock climber, but the techniques presented in this book have been **more valuable to me than anything I have ever worked at.**"
—Millerclmb, Carbondale, Il

"Pavel keeps delivering the goods. This book has the ingredients that you need to 'have wired in' if you want strength. Like all of Pavel's products, I wish I had this information when I was 20 years old. Better late, than never. **Four years of University with a double major in Phys Ed, it's not a patch on Pavel.**"
—Pete, Hobart, Australia

Excerpts from Customer Reviews Posted on www.dragondoor.com

"The program requires knowledge of only two exercises and a minimum of time. I have already tried the exercises. If you think bodyweight training is easy, you are in for a surprise. The book is well written and reads quickly. There are plenty of illustrations to help you understand the exercises involved. I look forward to incorporating Naked Warrior training to my routine. If you have bought from Dragon Door Publishing before, this book is the high quality product we have come to expect. For newcomers to the website, you won't be disappointed. For all who waited anxiously for Naked Warrior to arrive, it was worth the wait."
—Pat Cuntrera, Six Sigma Personal Training

"*The Naked Warrior* is a kick ass book! If you are looking to improve your strength, fitness level, learn some rock solid techniques that will take you to the next level of your game no matter what you do then The Naked Warrior is for you. I got the book because I saw Pavel perform the pistol squat in Muscle Media and wanted to know, "How the hell is that possible?" Practicing Pavel's techniques in *The Naked Warrior* I learned that it is possible because I can now do them.

My balance and leg strength is amazing after learning his secrets. I have improved my leg strength and sprinting power. His breathing and tension techniques I have also translated over to other parts of my workout which has led to improvement. I was most amazed when I got the attention of some pretty big body builders in my gym. Their jaws dropped as I performed weighted one-legged squats and they couldn't even perform one. This book isn't about getting massive but about pure strength!"
—M. Crandell

"The title doesn't really do this book justice. After reading the book a couple times, and practicing the techniques for increasing strength detailed in the book, I strict military pressed the 72lb kettlebell for the first time. The military press isn't even one of the drills in the book.

The body weight drills that are explored in such exacting detail in the book are great, and will allow you to build amazing strength without any weights whatsoever, but the real value lies in the principles in the book that apply to all strength training – period.

Just understanding how to "zip up" your body and pressurize your core will make you stronger on the spot. The chapter on Greasing the Groove will get you doing drills in a few weeks that look like circus tricks to you today. The details are explained in easy to understand terms, but don't let that fool you, this is high-end info. I'm down at the beach every weekend over the summer, last year I dragged my KBs with me every weekend, not this year - no need to. Get this book."
— Bill Fox

"Another great resource by Pavel on real world strength training. Everything you need to go from assisted 1-arm push-ups and Pistols to the real deal. Plus, instead of just doing the I say 'this I say that route' of most fitness books, Pavel showcases input from other Party member's on strength and conditioning.

This is a desert island classic. If confined with out KBs and or weights, this book and some 8-count bodybuilders would keep you hard."
—Dylan Thomas,RKC,Oku-iri Aki-Jujutsu

"*The Naked Warrior* is what most other books aspire to be. A down and dirty bare bones explanation about strength and strength dynamics in a no nonsense format.

While other books tell stories of how great those who contributed to it are, The Naked Warrior tells you how you can achieve the strength to take your fitness to the next level.

A little over a year ago, my exposure to Kettlebells was eye opening and has been a tremendous tool for my operational fitness, but now after 2 weeks using information from *The Naked Warrior* I have made even greater strides.

Since doing "grease the groove" for pistols and pullups, I have doubled the number of pistols I can do with the 24kg bell and have seen a marked improvement in my balance. I was able to do 2 pistols on a chain that was anchoring a vehicle and have done one while standing on the handle of my 32kg bell. I also have mastered the "true" one-armed push up.

I look forward to seeing more results as I improve on my "zip up" ability. *The Naked Warrior* will help to further increase the tactical advantage over the enemy."
— Counter Terrorist Operator

"The expansion on the tension-generation techniques first introduced in *Power ı The People* and on the power breathing techniques, is alone worth the price of the book. The context of these techniques, the bodyweight drills, also made me look at bodyweight training in a whole new light. It will be obvious to anyone who has seen Pavel's earlier works that these concepts have tremendous carryover to other physical activities such as lifting."
—**Paolo Valladolid**

"*The Naked Warrior* is the best thing I've ever read on strength training. Period. Although I already knew some of the ideas, the clarity of the presentation gave me a deeper understanding and therefore a better ability to apply them to my training. Many of the ideas were entirely new to me, and though they sounded reasonable, I needed to test them. I followed the directions to increase both my intra abdominal pressure and body tension. Surprisingly, although I'll need much practice to improve my techniques further, my one-arm chin is already noticeably stronger.

The Naked Warrior has increased my consciousness regarding the importance of technique. Shortly after reading it, I changed my training methods. I'm so excited because Naked Warrior has unleashed the power of my mind to contribute to my strength. It's not easy to teach an old dog new tricks, but Naked Warrior did just that.

I hesitated in getting *The Naked Warrior*, because one-arm pushups and pistols were not my thing. They are still not, but the strength building concepts were explained so well, that I was able to apply them to my goals."
— **Jack Arnow**

"If you are looking for a book containing scores of useless, half-baked exercise descriptions, do not buy this book. If you are interested in learning how to maximize your strength PERIOD, then this book is for you.

Pavel details every nuance of strength training through the dissection of two body weight drills. The astute reader will realize that these techniques are applicable to ANY strength training exercise, no matter is used to provide the resistance.

Pavel also details Grease the Groove, a powerful method for building strength through frequent practice.

Utilization of the techniques and careful self-examination of my one legged squat (Pistol) performance, has allowed me to begin performing them with the weight held in the racked position. Currently, I train with two 16 kg kettlebells racked, and two 24's are not far off.

In my opinion, *The Naked Warrior* is another "must read" from The Evil Russian. Thank you Pavel!"
—**David Finley**

The Naked Warrior

▼

Master the Secrets
of the Super-Strong
—Using Bodyweight Exercises Only

▲

By

Pavel

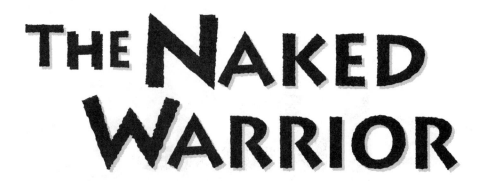

THE NAKED WARRIOR

▼

MASTER THE SECRETS
OF THE SUPER-STRONG
—USING BODYWEIGHT EXERCISES ONLY

Published in the United States by:
Dragon Door Publications, Inc
P.O. Box 4381, St. Paul, MN 55104
Tel: (651) 487-2180 • Fax: (651) 487-3954
Credit card orders: 1-800-899-5111
Email: dragondoor@aol.com • Website: www.dragondoor.com

ISBN: 0-938045-55-5

This edition first published in January 2004

Printed in the United States of America

Book design, Illustrations and cover by Derek Brigham
Website http//www.dbrigham.com
Tel/Fax: (612) 827-3431 • Email: dbrigham@visi.com
Photographs by Don Pitlik: (612) 252-6797

DISCLAIMER
The author and publisher of this material are not responsible in any manner whatsoever for any injury that may occur through following the instructions contained in this material. The activities, physical and otherwise, described herein for informational purposes only, may be too strenuous or dangerous for some people and the reader(s) should consult a physician before engaging in them.

DEDICATED

TO THE PARTY,
THE DRAGONDOOR.COM
STRENGTH FORUM

FOREWORD

"IT AIN'T NUTHIN' TILL I CALL IT."

Even if you're not a baseball fan, chances are that you've heard this quote by umpire Bill Klem. After reading *The Naked Warrior* those words took on new meaning for me. How many times have we seen someone perform a skill that appears to be magical? How many people do we know, or know of, who seem to be able to naturally do things that we can't do? The temptation is to shrug our shoulders and acknowledge their natural abilities, talents, and other inborn gifts. That is, until someone calls it. Until that someone can observe it, break it down, and describe it to the rest of us in a way that makes it possible for us to reproduce the "magic". That someone is Pavel. In his book, *The Naked Warrior*, Pavel presents us with a clear system for building a strong body that can perform acts of useful strength, the kind of strength that men have always needed to win when winning meant living another day.

I have spent my entire career instructing others, as a teacher, a coach and a trainer of bodies. One of things I do best is to shuffle my mental deck of exercise and technique cards and deal out new workouts. I am always adding to this deck because I have learned to be open to all sources of information and ideas. I take what I have read, heard or seen and sift it through the filters of more than three decades of education and experience. Then I try the result out on whoever is either unobservant enough to miss the "I've got something new" look in my eye, or brave enough not to care or slow enough not to escape in time. If it works, it goes in the deck.

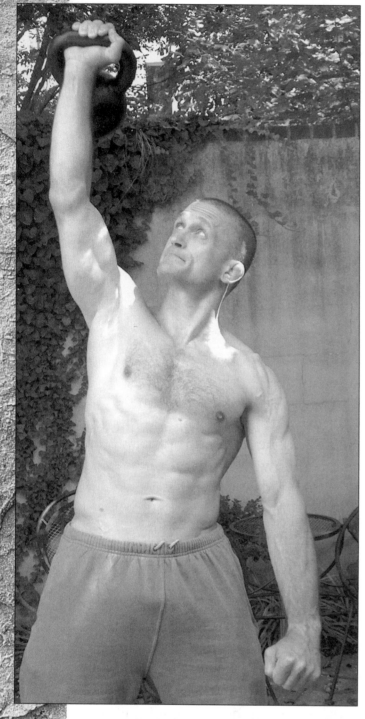

Steve Maxwell with the morning's military press

Pavel has been one of my most abundant sources of concepts and techniques that get into that deck. I sought him out after reading about Russian Kettlebell training, not realizing at the time what a broad contribution his work would be to my own. One of the biggest things that we share is a fundamental view of the vital connection that physical training has to performance in life, as well as sports. We are not so far removed as we think from strength and conditioning levels being essential for survival. One of the other things that we share is the outlook that superior strength and conditioning does not require sophisticated equipment, or a fashionable wardrobe, just some basic knowledge and a willingness to do the work.

I almost began this foreword with the quote "If you want to know why the racehorse runs fast, don't ask the horse." But I chose not use that particular quote because it doesn't apply to Pavel. Pavel is a racehorse who cannot only tell you exactly why a racehorse runs fast, but how you too can run like the racehorse. Pavel is a racehorse who can "call it". And he calls it in *The Naked Warrior.*

—*Steve Maxwell, MS, RKC Sr.,*
Brazilian Jiu-Jitsu World Champion,
Maxercise.com

TABLE OF CONTENTS

Chapter 1   7
The Naked Warrior Rules of Engagement

"The Naked Warrior", or why strength train with bodyweight?... **Strength. Pure strength**...the definition of strength...strength class-ifications ...examples of the three types of strength...the focus of The Naked Warrior...**The Naked Warrior rules of engagement**...the only way to build strength...high resistance and mental focus on contraction ...tension generation skill...the importance of "practice" over "workout"...a powerful instant-strength mix...**The Naked Warrior Principles**...the six keys to greater strength...**How do lifters really train?**..."best practice" secrets of powerlifters and Olympic weight lifters...**How do gymnasts get a good workout with the same weight?**...five strategies for making 5-rep exercises harder...how gymnasts achieve super strength...how to customize the resistance without changing the weight.

Chapter 2   21
The Naked Warrior Workout

"Grease the groove," or how to get superstrong without a routine...the secret success formula...**Some GTG testimonials from the dragondoor .com forum**...how does the GTG system work?...turning your nerves into superconductors...avoiding muscle failure...strength as a skill—the magic formula... **"The Pistol": the Russian Spec Ops' leg strengthener of choice**...rate yourself against the Russian hard guys...how to do it—the basics...doing fewer exercises better...**The one-arm/one-leg pushup: "an exercise in total body tension"**...what gymnastics has to teach us...another advantage of the one-arm pushup...GTG, the ultimate specialization program.

Chapter 3   35
High-Tension Techniques for Instant Strength

Tension. What force is made of…the relationship between tension and force…high-tension techniques…**"Raw strength" versus "technique"** …the power of mental focus…**Low gear for brute force**…speed and tension …putting explosiveness in context…**"Doesn't dynamic tension act like a brake?"**…a dirty little secret of bodybuilding…the dangers of mindless lifting…**The power of a fist**…the principle of irradiation …**Accidental discharge of strength: a tip from firearms instructors** …interlimb response and your muscle software…**Power abs = a power body**…the relationship between abs tension and body strength…why flat abs are strong abs and sucked in waists are weak…the "back-pressure crunch"…**Put your "rear-wheel drive" in high gear**…the source of real striking power…the handgrip test…**A gymnast instantly gains 40 pounds of strength on his iron cross with the three techniques you have just learned**…**The "static stomp": using ground pressure to maximize power**…**Tense your lats and keep your shoulders down: a secret of top karatekas and bench pressers**…how the secret of armpit power translates into paydirt for one-arm pushups, punches, and bench presses…**"The corkscrew": Another secret of the karate punch**…the power of rotation and spiral…the invisible force…**Bracing: boost your strength up to 20% with an armwrestling tactic**…when to brace…the advantage of dead-start exercises…**"Body hardening"—tough love for teaching tension**…the quick and hard way to greater tension control…**Beyond bracing: "zipping up"**…taking your pretensing skills to a new level…**Wind up for power**…the art of storing elastic energy for greater power…the reverse squat.

Chapter 4   73
Power Breathing: The Martial Arts Masters' Secret for Superstrength

Bruce Lee called it "breath strength"…cranking up your breath strength…your body as a first-class sound system—how to make it happen…definition of true power breathing…**Power inhalation**…the mystery breathing muscle that's vital to your strength…amping up the compression…when and why to hold your breath…**Reverse power breathing: evolution of the Iron Shirt technique**…the pelvic diaphragm lock…to crucial rules for maximal power breathing…**Power up from the core, or the "pneumatics of Chi"**…two important principles of power generation…how to avoid a power leakage…the "balloon" technique for greater power.

Chapter 5   91
Driving GTG Home

Driving GTG home: focused…skill-building—why "fewer is better" …the law of the jungle…**Driving GTG home: flawless**…how to achieve perfection—the real key…the five conditions for generating high tension…the significance of low rep work…**Driving GTG home: frequent**…the one great secret of press success…**Driving GTG home: fresh**…the many aspects of staying fresh for optimal strength gains…staying away from failure…the balancing act between frequency and freshness…**Driving GTG home: fluctuating**…how to avoid training plateaus…**"same yet different"** strategies…"waviness of load" …countering fatigue…training guidelines for a PR…backing off and overtraining…**Summing up GTG**…**Summing up GTG even more**… compressing GTG in ten words or less.

Chapter 6   103
Field-Stripping the Pistol

Box Pistol…how to go from zero to hero…the box squat—a champions' favorite for multi-muscle strength gains…making a quantum leap in your squats…various options from easier to eviler…the rocking pistol…how to recruit your hip flexors…how to avoid cramping…**One-Legged Squat, Paul Anderson style…Airborne Lunge…Pistol Classic**…mastering the real deal…**Negative-Free Pistol**…the three advantages of concentric-only training…**Renegade Pistol…Fire-in-the-Hole Pistol…Cossack Pistol… Dynamic Isometric Pistol**…combining dynamic exercise with high-tension stops…multiple stops for greater pain…taking advantage of your sticking points…easier variations…three reasons why adding isos to dynamic lifting can increase effectiveness by up to 15%…protecting yourself against injury…**Isometric Pistol**…holding tension over time…the art of "powered-down" high-tension techniques…**Weighted Pistol**…working the spinal erectors.

Chapter 7   151
Field-Stripping the One-Arm Pushup

The One-Arm Pushup, floor and elevated...how to shine at high-intensity exertion...change-ups for easy and difficult...the authorized technique ...developing a controlled descent...Isometric One-Arm Pushup...The One-Arm Dive Bomber Pushup...The One-Arm Pump...The One-Arm Half Bomber Pushup...Four more drills to work up to the One-Arm Dive Bomber...The One-Arm/One-Leg Pushup...the Tsar of the one-arm pushups.

Chapter 8   173
Naked Warrior Q&A

Are bodyweight exercises superior to exercises with weights?...the advantage of cals...what cals enforce...the biggest disadvantage of bodyweight exercising...the advantage of barbells...the advantages and disadvantages of dumbbells...the advantages of kettlebells...**Why is there such an intense argument in the martial arts community as to whether bodyweight exercises are superior to exercises with weights?**...confusions explained...what a fighter needs...**Can I get very strong using only bodyweight exercises?**...**Should I mix different strength-training tools in my training?**...**How can I incorporate bodyweight exercises with kettlebell and barbell training?**...**Can the high-tension techniques and GTG system be applied to weights?**... **Can the high-tension techniques and GTG system be applied to strength endurance training?**...**I can't help overtraining. What should I do?**...**Can I follow the Naked Warrior program on an ongoing basis?**...**Can I add more exercises to the Naked Warrior program?**...**Will my development be unbalanced from doing only two exercises?**...**Is there a way to work the lats with a pulling exercise when no weights or pullup bars are accessible?**...door pullups ...door rows...**Where can I learn more about bodyweight-only strength training?**...**Low reps and no failure? This training is too easy!**...**Will I forget all the strength techniques in some sort of emergency?**...**Isn't dedicating most of the book to technique too much?**...why technique is crucial...moving from ordinary to extraordinary...**Parting shot**...there are no excuses!

CHAPTER ONE

THE NAKED WARRIOR RULES OF ENGAGEMENT

- "The Naked Warrior", or why strength train with bodyweight?
- Strength. Pure strength.
- The Naked Warrior rules of engagement
- How do lifters really train?
- How do gymnasts get a good workout with the same weight?

"The Naked Warrior", or why strength train with bodyweight?

Because it is always there.

Tony Blauer*, one of the top defensive tactics and close-quarter combat instructors in the law enforcement and military communities, coined the expression "a Naked Warrior". "I should be able to take care of myself even

* For more information on Tony Blauer see the back of this book.

if I am naked," says Blauer. "But it goes without saying that I will do better with an MP5, a Kevlar vest, and a good S.W.A.T. team."

The same principle applies to strength training. You will make your best gains if you have access to quality hardware: barbells, kettlebells, pullup bars, and so on. But, unless you live the predictable life of a greenhouse plant, sooner or later you will end up in a situation in which you have no iron around.

Refuse to cave in to the circumstances.

Being able to improvise something out of nothing is a skill highly valued by the Russian Special Forces. Do you know how to wash yourself with ashes from a bonfire? Can you keep your feet warm by stuffing dry grass inside your foot wraps? Can you rig up a time bomb out of a hand grenade and a cigarette?

Can you get a quality strength workout anywhere, anytime?

Now you can.

Quoting Theodore Roosevelt, "Do what you can, with what you have, where you are."

Strength. Pure strength.

You cannot be 'just strong'. The idiotic question, "Who is stronger, powerlifters or strongmen?" can be compared to "Who will win in a fight, a shark or a lion?" On land or in the water?

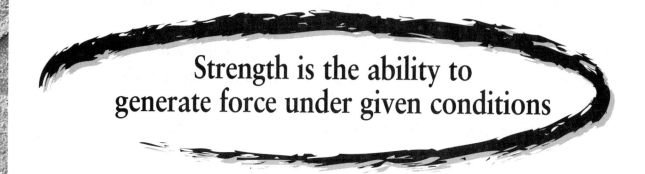

Strength is the ability to
generate force under given conditions

Strength can mean a lot of different things. It cannot be taken out of context.

Strength is defined as the ability to generate force *under given conditions*.

Here is a highly simplified, in the trenches, classification of strength:

maximal strength,
explosive strength, and
strength endurance.

Russian Kyokushinkai full-contact karate fighter and instructor Oleg Ignatov gives the following examples of bodyweight drills that develop these three types of strength:

- **Pushups:** the one-arm pushup (max strength), the clapping pushup (explosive strength), and the repetition pushup (strength endurance)
- **Squats:** the one-legged squat (max strength), low-rep vertical and broad jumps (explosive strength), vertical and broad jumps for up to 50 reps (strength endurance), repetition squats (strength endurance)

The focus of *The Naked Warrior* is max strength, period.

Why?

- Because pure strength gets very little attention in popular books— obsessed as they are with the high-rep pump.
- Because enough has already been said about strength endurance.
- Because, for a long time, your explosive strength will automatically increase along with your max strength.
- Because what you look like has no bearing on what you can do.

Power to you!

9

The Naked Warrior Rules of Engagement

If you were looking for another mindless routine of repetition pushups and situps to pump yourself up, you have come to the wrong place. *The Naked Warrior* is about strength—period.

A hard man with no access to weights cannot afford a high-rep compromise.

It is a fact: respectable strength can only be built with high-resistance, low-rep exercises that impose high levels of tension on the muscles.

Note that I said 'resistance', not 'weight'. A case in point: There are a lot more double-bodyweight benchers out there than men who can chin themselves with one arm.

The Naked Warrior will show you how to make select bodyweight drills so challenging you will only be able to squeeze out a couple of reps. You will do this by altering the leverage and weight distribution between the limbs. If pushups are easy for you, then do them on one arm. If you are a stud and one-armers are no problem, then elevate your feet. You get the picture. By the same token, calisthenics (or cals) can be customized to be made easier. For instance, do one-arm pushups with your hands elevated, rather than your feet.

It is an axiom in serious strength training with iron that the best gains are made by focusing on a limited number of high-resistance, full-body exercises, such as deadlifts and snatches. The Naked Warrior program features only two anywhere-anytime drills: the one-legged squat and the one-arm pushup. These exercises are brutally hard and work the whole body. They are the bodyweight equivalents of the powerlifts.

Strength is built by tensing the muscles harder, not by exhausting them with countless reps.

High resistance is one of the two requirements of high tension. The other is mental focus on contracting the muscles harder. The tension-generating skill is the most important variable in getting stronger—much more important than muscle mass. If this were not true, Alexey Sivokon would not have benched 500 pounds at 148 pounds of bodyweight and matching height.

Since strength is a skill, training must be approached as a 'practice', not a 'workout'. Thus, the Naked Warrior routine is unlike any other you have seen. You will practice every day, throughout the day; you will focus on max tension; and you will totally avoid muscle fatigue and failure. Strength gains will come fast and furious.

"I went from 5 to 10 pullups in one week," reported 235-pound Chris Rubio, RKC, on the dragondoor.com forum. His gains are not unusual.

Another distinctive feature of the Naked Warrior program is the high-tension techniques. Simply tensing the target muscles hard is great, but you can contract them even harder—much harder—by applying ancient martial arts tension secrets. *The Naked Warrior* has systematized them into a powerful instant-strength mix.

Jeff Selleg, Valley SRT Training/Operations Officer with the Port of Seattle Police, wrote, "Pavel, thanks for the training at the ASLET [American Society of Law Enforcement Training] conference. I am completely sold on your techniques. After your three-hour seminar, I added six pullups." How can such quick gains be possible? Through increasing the intensity of the muscular contraction.

Power to you, Naked Warrior! Anywhere. Anytime.

The Naked Warrior Principles

- Strength is built by tensing the muscles harder, not by exhausting them with reps.
- High tension requires high resistance and mental focus on contracting the muscles harder.
- High resistance can be achieved without heavy weights by deliberately imposing poor leverage and unfavorable weight distribution between the limbs.
- The best strength gains are made by focusing on a limited number of high-resistance, low-rep, full-body exercises. The Naked Warrior program features only two exercises: the one-legged squat and the one-arm pushup. They are the bodyweight equivalents of the powerlifts.
- Strength is a skill. Training must be approached as a practice, not a workout. You will practice every day, throughout the day; you will focus on

max tension; and you will totally avoid muscle fatigue and failure.

- The skill of tension-generation is the most important variable in getting stronger—it is much more important than the building of muscle mass.
- The martial arts high-tension techniques will make you stronger by enabling you to tense your muscles harder.

How do lifters really train?

A book on max strength training—and when it comes down to it, it makes no difference whether you are lifting a barbell or your own body—would not be complete without tipping a hat to the people who have made strength their only pursuit: Olympic weightlifters and powerlifters.

How do these specialists train? If you don't belong to this exclusive community, chances are that you lump together lifters and bodybuilders into the same category and presume they follow the same "do or die" reps-to-failure shtick. Nothing could be further from the truth.

A limited number of exercises, mostly the two competition lifts and their variations, done in 6 to 10 sets of 1 to 3 reps each is the classic Olympic weightlifting blueprint for strength. Powerlifters follow a similar schedule, although their reps climb up to 5 and even 6 because the powerlifts are not as technically demanding as the snatch and the C&J. Powerlifters tend to do fewer sets because the deadlifts are more exhausting than the snatches.

Weightlifters train almost daily, often twice or even three times a day. Many powerlifters still practice each lift once a week, but this practice is quickly becoming obsolete. It's hard to ignore the fact that the victorious Russian men's national powerlifting team benches up to 8 times a week.

Neither group trains to failure. Weightlifters don't do more than 3 reps even with half their max. Powerlifters are the same way. The great ones rack the bar with at least a rep or two in the bank, unless they are in a meet.

Both breeds of strength athlete know that training continually with the same intensity or volume will flatline their strength gains. So, they play the game of "two steps forward, one step back": first pushing ahead and then backing off.

Lifters practice the generation of greater tension relentlessly. Bench press record breaker George Halbert crushes the bar to pulp. World champion powerlifter Ernie Frantz practiced tensing up his whole body throughout the day. World record squatter Dr. Judd Biasiotto visualized tensing his muscles in the perfect sequence for each lift.

Once you strip away the drama and demagoguery, strength building, whether with your body or with iron, is simple and straightforward:

Engage a skeleton crew of full body exercises; **perform** multiple sets of up to 5 reps—never going to failure and with plenty of rest between sets; **employ** total focus on technique and tension; and **vary** volume and intensity continuously.

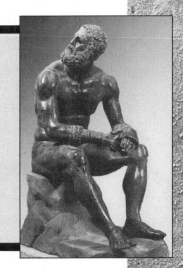

HOW LIFTERS REALLY TRAIN

- Limited number of 'big' exercises
- Multiple sets of up to 5 reps, never to failure and with plenty of rest between sets
- Total focus on technique and tension
- Continuous variation in volume and intensity

You are about to learn how these principles can be successfully applied to strength training with a limited, unchanging weight—yours.

How do gymnasts get a good workout with the same weight?

NOT by mindlessly adding reps. "...endless pushups, sit-ups or, for the strong, perhaps pull-ups and dips," says Christopher Sommer, a gymnastics coach from Desert Devils in Phoenix, AZ, are "great maybe for general fitness or endurance, but of little value in building real strength."

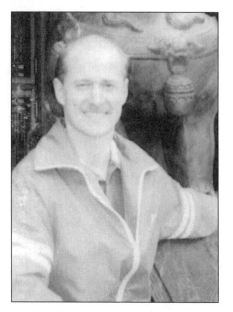

Christopher Sommer has coached state, regional, and national gymnastics champions. To schedule a seminar e-mail him at olympicbodies@aol.com.

Performing more than 6 reps per set hinders strength development, insists Arkady Vorobyev, a leading Russian sports scientist and former world champion weightlifter. Robert Roman, another top gun of Russian weightlifting, explains that muscular tension or weight builds strength, rather than fatigue or reps. He clarifies that doing more reps generates less tension than exerting a brief maximal or near-maximal effort. So, if you expect to get stronger in the bench press or the one-arm pushup by knocking off 100 pushups, you have got another thing coming. And no, there is nothing magical or mysterious about your bodyweight versus iron that suddenly changes all the laws of strength training.

> There is nothing magical or mysterious about your bodyweight versus iron that suddenly changes all the laws of strength training.

The question is:

If we have only so many pounds of weight to work with, how can we make the exercise hard enough in 6 reps or less?

Simple:

By **redistributing your weight between your limbs, manipulating the range of motion, training in an unstable environment, varying the leverage, and minimizing bounce and momentum.**

Let's consider these strategies one at a time.

Redistribute your weight between your limbs

When you do a basic floor pushup, your weight is distributed between your hands and your feet, say, 50/50. Elevate your feet on a bench and you will be pushing up 70 percent of your bodyweight. Lift your feet even higher and you will get an 80/20 distribution. Go up in a handstand and you will be lifting 100 percent (or almost 100 percent—your forearms will stay put).

You get the idea. The opposite principle also holds true. Rest your hands on a desk or even a wall and you will be pushing up but a fraction of your weight.

Another example of weight redistribution is doing a two-arm pushup but shifting more weight to one arm. Keep unloading one arm more and more as you get stronger, until you are doing a legit one-arm pushup. Lifting one leg up is another option.

Helping yourself up with your hands while doing one-legged squats inside a doorway is another way to manipulate the weight distribution.

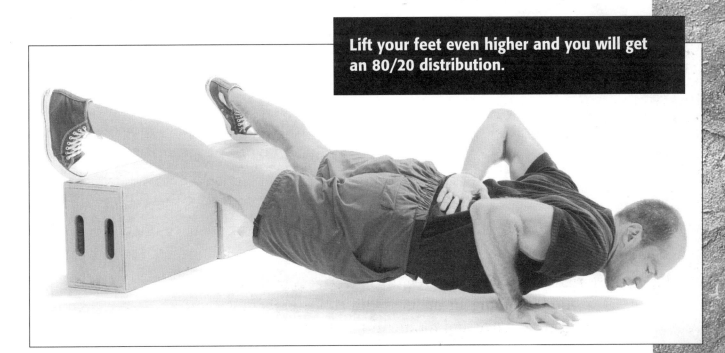

Lift your feet even higher and you will get an 80/20 distribution.

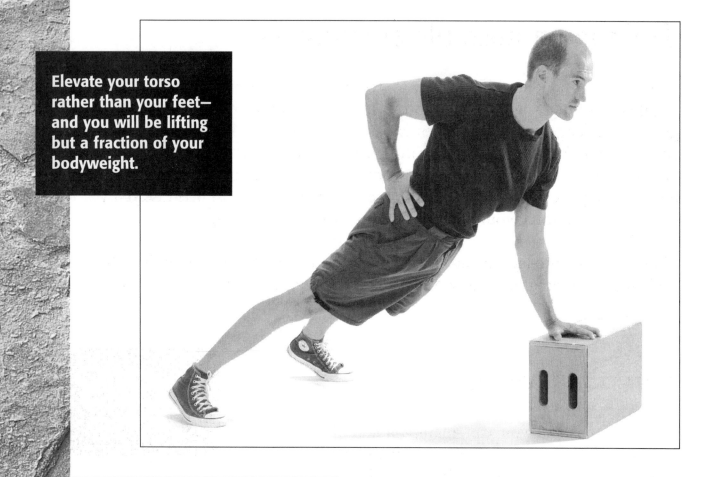

Elevate your torso rather than your feet— and you will be lifting but a fraction of your bodyweight.

Manipulate the range of motion

Redistributing your weight is the primary approach to resistance variation you will use with the Naked Warrior drills, but it is not the only one. You will also be manipulating your range of motion in some drills. A butt-to-the-floor one-legged squat, as favored by the Russian Special Forces, may be in your distant future, but I am sure you can sit down on a tall bench and come up on one leg.

I am sure you can sit down on a tall bench and come up on one leg.

16

Train in an unstable environment

Strength is about tension. One way to amp the tension is to use heavier weights—but that's not an option in this program. Another way to provide a greater challenge to your muscles is to perform an exercise in an unstable environment. Armed forces powerlifting champion Jack Reape has taught me an interesting variation of the decline pushup: Instead of putting your feet up on a bench, park them on top of the handles of two kettlebells. The instability of the bells will force your entire body to stay tight and strong.

The one-arm/one-legged pushup featured in this book also multiplies the challenge by adding instability. So does the one-legged squat.

Vary the leverage

Another variable you can manipulate is the leverage. The ancient Greek scientist and mathematician Archimedes bragged that he could tip the world with a lever that was sufficiently long—and he had a point. But leverage works both ways. By reducing it, an exercise can be made harder. The iron cross on the rings is not even in the same ballpark with pullups when it comes to difficulty, even though both involve lifting exactly the same amount of weight.

Practicing with an extreme lack of leverage is one of the secrets to gymnasts' super strength. "The name of the game is resistance," says Chris Sommer in the excerpt from his upcoming book *Building the Olympic Body,* posted on the articles, page of dragondoor.com. "A muscle contracts against resistance and, with perseverance, over time, becomes stronger. For strength to increase, the amount of resistance, or load worked against, must also increase over

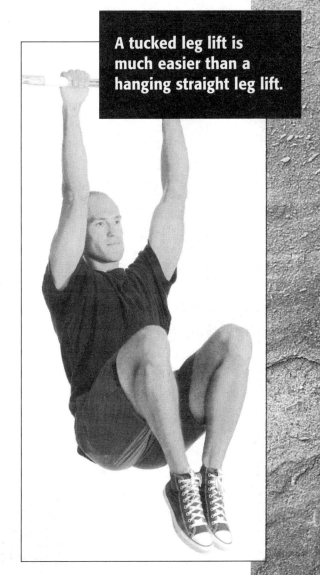

A tucked leg lift is much easier than a hanging straight leg lift.

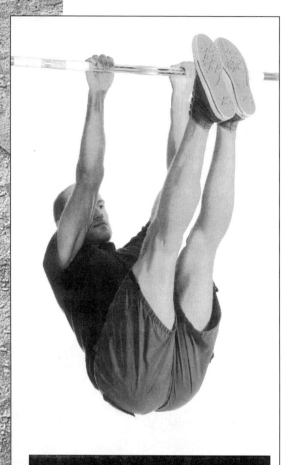

By straightening the legs, we have effectively doubled the difficulty of the exercise.

time. Hence the problem with bodyweight conditioning. When the resistance (the weight of the body) is fixed, how can you continue to increase strength? The answer is surprisingly simple—by decreasing the amount of leverage it is possible to exert on an exercise, the resistance of an exercise becomes increasingly greater. For example, a hanging straight leg lift is much harder than a tucked leg lift. In both exercises, the weight of your legs remains constant; however, by reducing your leverage (i.e., in this case, straightening your legs), we are able to greatly increase the resistance. By straightening the legs, we have effectively doubled the difficulty of the exercise, even though the weight of the body has remained constant."

Here is an interesting approach to manipulating leverage. In *Pull Your Own Weight*, Rick Osbourne and Brian McCaskey recommend 'pivot point variation', "which refers to the age old technique of dropping your knees to the ground in order to reduce the load in a push up. With the old standard method, you have two potential pivot points:

1) your knees, and 2) your feet. And, strangely enough, it can be a long ways from your knees to your feet when you're ready to make progress... simply use a small bench that can be placed under your body at any point between your hips and your feet. When the bench is moved toward your hips, resistance is reduced. As your strength increases, the bench should gradually be moved toward your toes. Eventually, of course, the idea is to eliminate the PPV bench altogether..."

Say no to the bounce and momentum

You can also increase the difficulty of bodyweight exercises by minimizing bounce and momentum. There are two ways of doing this.

The first is 'dead starts'. Using the one-arm pushup example, you would not touch your chest to the deck and go. You will lie down and totally relax on the deck, then flex again and power back up.

The second technique is dynamic isometrics. It involves pausing for a few seconds and staying tight at the sticking points of the exercise before moving along. Going back to the one-arm pushup example, you pause for 1 to 5 seconds with your chest almost touching the deck. Pain is good!

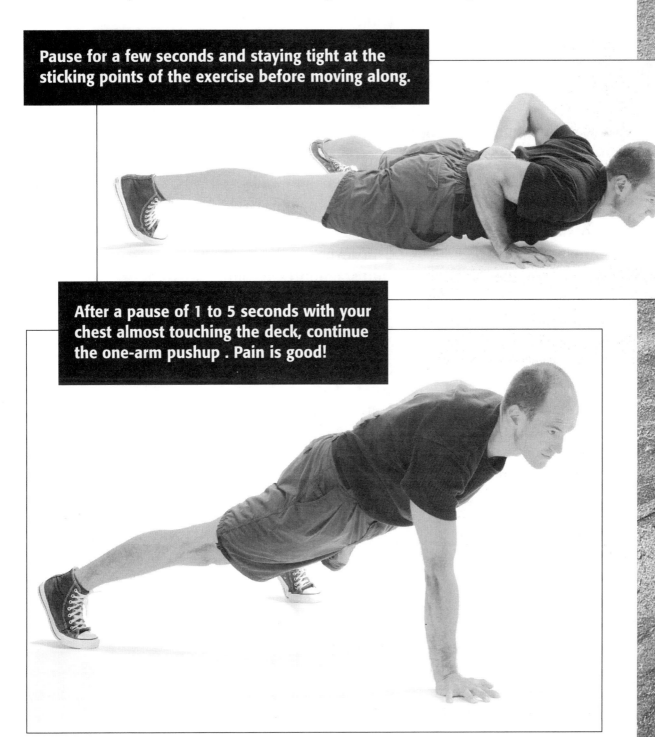

Pause for a few seconds and staying tight at the sticking points of the exercise before moving along.

After a pause of 1 to 5 seconds with your chest almost touching the deck, continue the one-arm pushup . Pain is good!

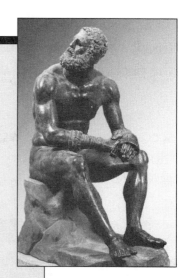

HOW TO CUSTOMIZE THE RESISTANCE WITHOUT CHANGING THE WEIGHT

- Redistribute your weight between your limbs
- Manipulate the range of motion
- Train in an unstable environment
- Vary the leverage
- Say no to the bounce and momentum

Christopher Sommer concludes, "With experience and creativity, it is possible to learn or design exercises that, done correctly and with the proper progressions, are so lacking in leverage that even at bodyweight levels of resistance, it is possible to build staggering amounts of strength."

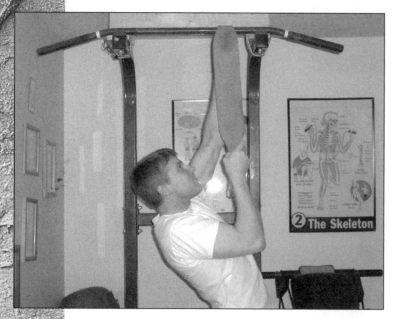

Former gymnast Brad Johnson demonstrates that the sky is the limit when using a variety of bodyweight strength exercises. *Photo courtesy Brad Johnson*

CHAPTER TWO

THE NAKED WARRIOR WORKOUT

- "Grease the groove," or how to get superstrong without a routine
- "The Pistol": The Russian Spec Ops' leg strengthener of choice
- The one-arm/one-leg pushup: "An exercise in total body tension"

"Grease the groove," or how to get superstrong without a routine

This program was first published in MILO: A Journal for Serious Strength Athletes. I insist that you subscribe to this top-quality publication at ironmind.com.

Our communist enemies who are trying to bury us have exercise breaks instead of coffee breaks.
—Bob Hoffman, York Barbell Club

Once, I came across this question posted on a popular strength-training website by a young Marine: "How should I train to improve my pullups?"

I was amused when I read the arcane and nonspecific advice the trooper received: "Do straight-arm pulldowns, reverse curls, avoiding the negative part of the chin-up every third workout..."

I had a radical thought:

If you want to get good at pullups, why not try to do...a lot of pullups?

Just a couple of months earlier, I had put my father-in-law, Roger Antonson, incidentally an ex-Marine, on a program that required him to do an easy 5 chins every time he went down to his basement. Each day, he would total between 25 and a 100 chinups, hardly breaking a sweat. Every month or so Roger would take a few days off and then test himself. Before you knew it, the old leatherneck could knock off 20 consecutive chins, more than he could do 40 years ago as a young jarhead!

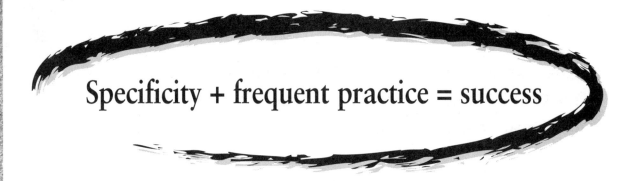

Specificity + frequent practice = success

A few months later, Roger sold his house and moved into an apartment. Being the paranoid Red that I am, I suspected that he plotted to work around the "chin every time you go to the basement" clause in his program. By Politburo decree, Comrade Antonson was issued one of those "Door Gym" pullup bars. He wisely conceded to the will of the Party and carried on with his "grease the chin-up groove" program.

My father, Vladimir, a Soviet Army officer, had me follow an identical GTG routine in my early testosterone years. My parents' apartment had a built-in storage space above the kitchen door. (This is a Russian design—you wouldn't understand.) Every time I left the kitchen, I would hang on to the ledge and crank out as many fingertip pullups as I could without struggling.

Consequently, my high school pullup tests were a breeze. (FYI: In Russian high schools, boys must do 12 strict palms over pullups to ace the test, and they fail if they do anything under 8.)

According to the conventional bodybuilding wisdom, Roger and I could not possibly have gotten stronger following this program. Training a muscle more than a couple of times a week is 'overtraining'! And where is the intensity?

But we did. And so did countless Russians and many Americans after I wrote this program up a few years ago in *MILO: A Journal for Serious Strength Athletes*. Here are but a few of the many testimonials you can find on the dragondoor.com discussion site.

Some GTG Testimonials from the dragondoor.com Forum

GTG Rocks!

From: Conrad • Date/Time 2002-05-16 01:14:43

I did a week of GTG with pistols and handstand pushups. At the beginning, I could do 1 wobbly pistol with my left leg—1 to a first stair step with my right, and 2 handstand pushups. By the end of the week, I was cranking 2 with each leg and 2 HSPUs [handstand pushups] throughout the day. Today, after about a week off, I tried again and did 5 clean ass-to-ground pistols with each leg and 5 HSPUs! Thanks, Pavel and the Party, for programs that work! Now I'll have to start adding weight and ROM.

Fastest hypertrophy ever on GTG?

From: Rocko • Date/Time 2002-09-12 18:47:54

While working to strengthen my calves to take more stress and allow myself to run properly, I've been doing GTG unweighted calf raises. In 7 days, I've gone from not being able to see anything when I flexed it to having it extend a half inch out the sides of the other muscles in my legs and seeing the whole thing like an anatomy chart, from back of knee to Achilles tendon. It shocked me today when I flexed my calves just to look and see what was going on. GTG works! :)

I went from 5 to 10 [pullups at 235 pounds of bodyweight] in 1 week following GTG

From: Chris Rubio, RKC • Date/Time 2003-04-23 21:33:22

MORE GTG TESTIMONIALS

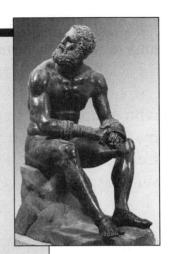

8-week GTG pullup results

From: runc2 • Date/Time 2003-04-13 13:38:05

When I started doing GTG for pullups 8 weeks ago, I could do only 1 assisted pullup. Today I maxed with 6 dead-hang pullups!

Two max rep PRs...

From: Eric Bruesch • Date/Time 2003-08-27 13:08:18

Last night, I did . . . 15 one-armed pushups each arm. Two months ago, I could not do one complete rep. GTG practice is 100% responsible for the progress . .

How does the GTG system work?

By literally greasing the groove for your chosen exercise.

Your technique will become so good from doing so many submaximal sets (in other words, from practicing) that once you decide to go all out, more 'nerve force' will reach your muscles because your nerves will have become superconductors.

The result? A PR (personal record), even though you will never have come close to your limit in training!

This will seem counterintuitive, if you are in the old workout mode. But it will make perfect sense, once you approach your strength training as practice.

It is critical for the program's success that you avoid muscle failure. Do not come even close to failure, whether you train for max or reps!

A good guideline is to do half the reps you could do if you put your heart into it (although there is nothing wrong with doing even fewer reps). Roger Antonson had worked up to training sets of 9 by the time he set a personal record of 20 chinups.

Since the Naked Warrior program is aimed at pure strength, do 5 reps max and select harder variations of the bodyweight exercises.

Strength is a skill. Professor Vladimir Zatsiorsky, a Soviet strength expert who jumped ship to America from the Dark Side, has summed up this notion by saying that an athlete must "do as much work as possible while being as fresh as possible." If you have a hard time remembering this best ever summary of effective strength training, get it tattooed on your arm.

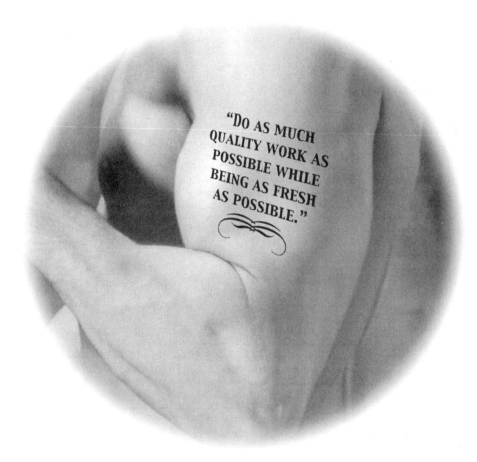

"The Pistol": The Russian Spec Ops' leg strengthener of choice

If you want to develop strong legs and have no resistance to work with but your bodyweight, there is only one exercise that will deliver:

The one-legged squat, which we fondly called "the pistol" in the Russian *Spetsnaz*. Just go rock bottom on one leg, holding your other nearly straight out in front, and then get up without bouncing. No sweat, right?

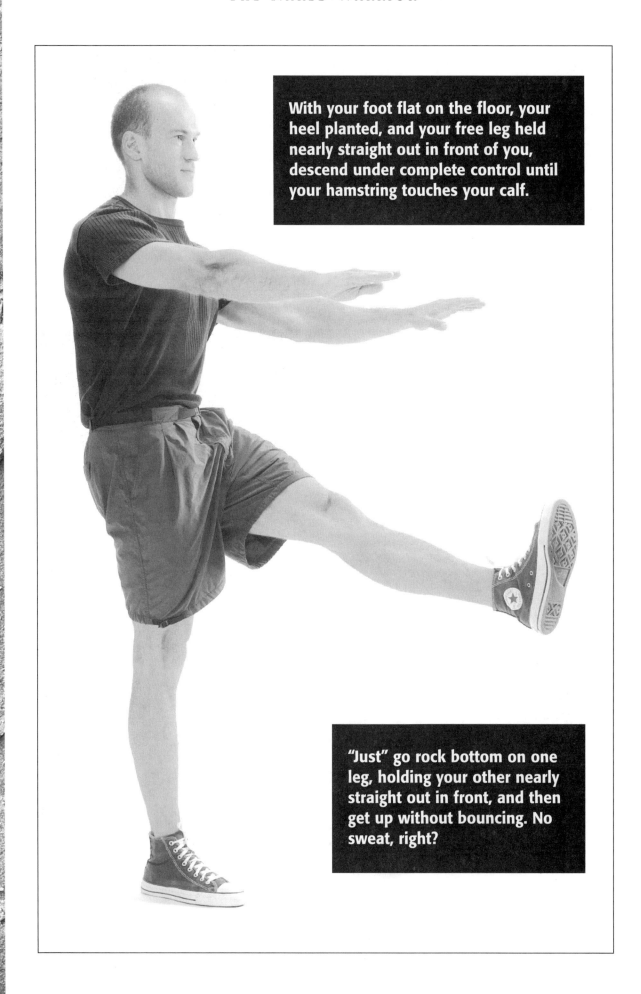

With your foot flat on the floor, your heel planted, and your free leg held nearly straight out in front of you, descend under complete control until your hamstring touches your calf.

"Just" go rock bottom on one leg, holding your other nearly straight out in front, and then get up without bouncing. No sweat, right?

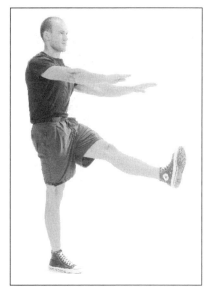

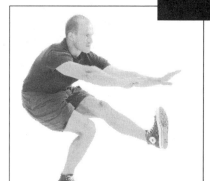

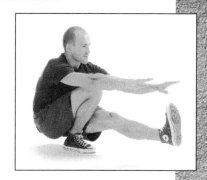

Do not bounce.

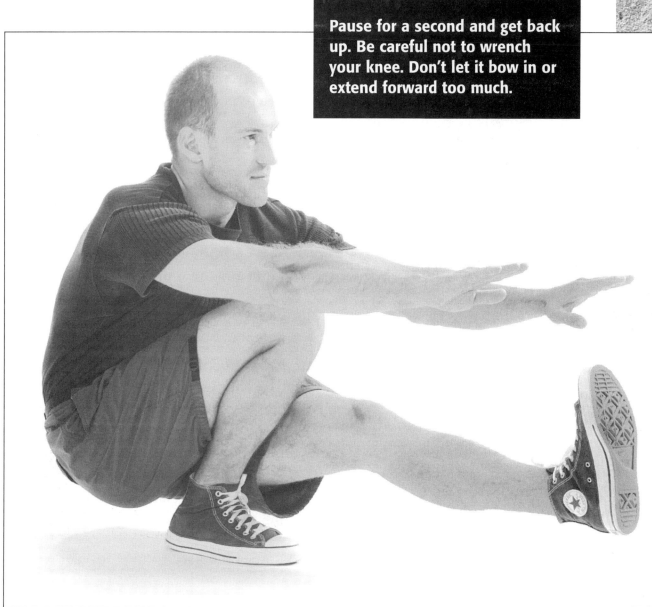

Pause for a second and get back up. Be careful not to wrench your knee. Don't let it bow in or extend forward too much.

Do you want to know how you rate against an everyday Russian hard guy?

According to the battery of PT tests developed by S. Lobanov and A. Chumakov, Masters of Sports of the All-Union Research Institute in Russia, 10 consecutive pistols per leg are "satisfactory," 15 are "good," and 20 are "excellent." You should be able to work up to 20 without ever doing more than 5 in training. Just make them harder and harder by adding pauses, kettlebells, and so on.

Time to get down to business. With your foot flat on the floor, your heel planted, and your free leg held nearly straight out in front of you, descend under complete control until your hamstring touches your calf. Do not bounce; pause for a second and get back up. Be careful not to wrench your knee. Don't let it bow in or extend forward too much.

If you can pull off a clean pistol following these instructions (which are typical in scope, or rather lack thereof, for strength-training books), then my hat is off to you. But I think you will not. My point is this: Do fewer exercises and pay attention to details. Street fighters who have polished one or two moves always dominate black belts who know 10 ways to block a punch.

Later in this book, you will find a comprehensive step-by-step guide for taking your one-legged squats (or pistols) and one-arm pushups (the *only* exercises in the Naked Warrior program) from zero to hero—plus many cool

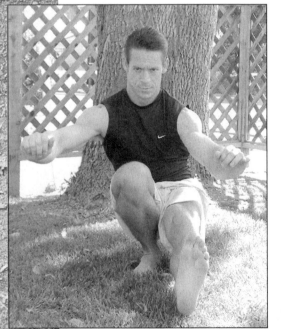

variations that are both harder and easier than regular pistols and one-arm pushups.

You can do a lot of things and be mediocre or you can achieve amazing heights through laser-like focus. National full-contact kung fu champion Steve Cotter, RKC Sr., worked up to 80 consecutive one-legged squats while still in his teens! (In case you don't know, 'RKC' stands for 'Russian Kettlebell Challenge' and denotes a certified instructor. The 'Sr.' designation means Steve is one of a handful of elite senior instructors.

National full-contact kung fu champion Steve Cotter, RKC Sr., has done 80 consecutive bodyweight pistols per leg and 14 pistols with a 72 lb. kettlebell, and a rep with two 72 lb kettlebells. Laser like focus pays off. *Photo courtesy fullkontactkettlebells.com.*

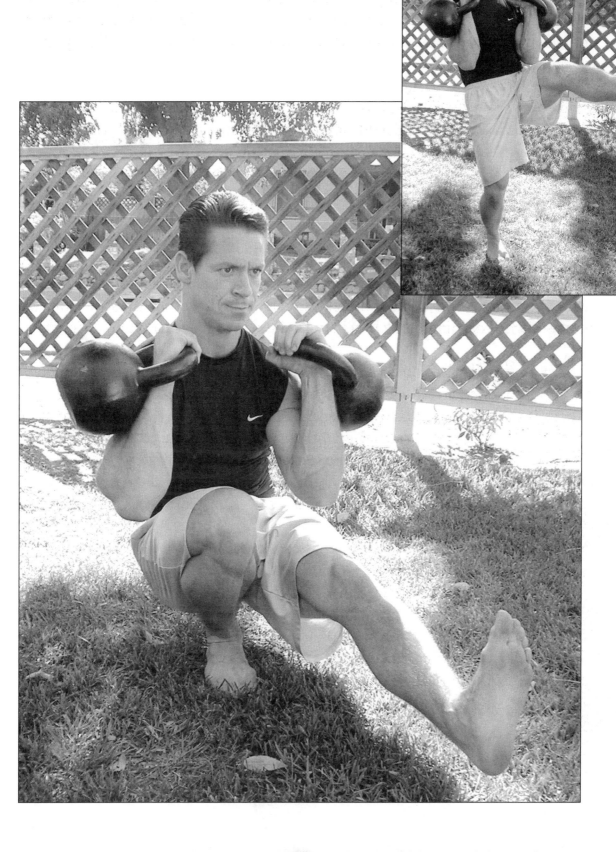

"I fractured my wrist playing catch on the blacktop with a football..." recalls Cotter, the owner of FullKOntactKettlebells.com. "When others [at my martial arts school] did pushups, I did pistols. When they did hand-whipping drills, I did pistols. It got to a point where when the class was doing a set of pushups, I was matching them 1 for 1 with pistols. So it was kind of by mistake, and through training around an injury, that it warranted doing enough practice of the exercise to get really effortless and comfortable with it."

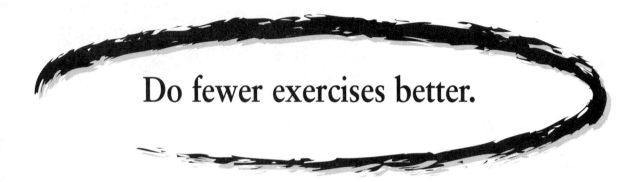

Do fewer exercises better.

The one-arm/one-leg pushup: "An exercise in total body tension"

"It is a mistake to think that Physical Training becomes more satisfactory and attractive according to the number of exercises used," wrote K.A. Knudsen, chief instructor of gymnastics for Denmark in his 1920 *A Textbook of Gymnastics*. "The teacher of gymnastics must learn the art of limiting himself. Far too often the short time given in the school curriculum to Physical Training is wasted on exercises of little value. Therefore the first thing required of a teacher of gymnastics is that he should be capable of estimating the value of the exercises he uses."

The one-arm/one-leg pushup is such an exercise.

Note that your shoulders must stay parallel to the floor, your chest must almost touch the floor, and your foot may not be resting on its edge but on the ball.

This move is much more than a stunt to impress your friends.

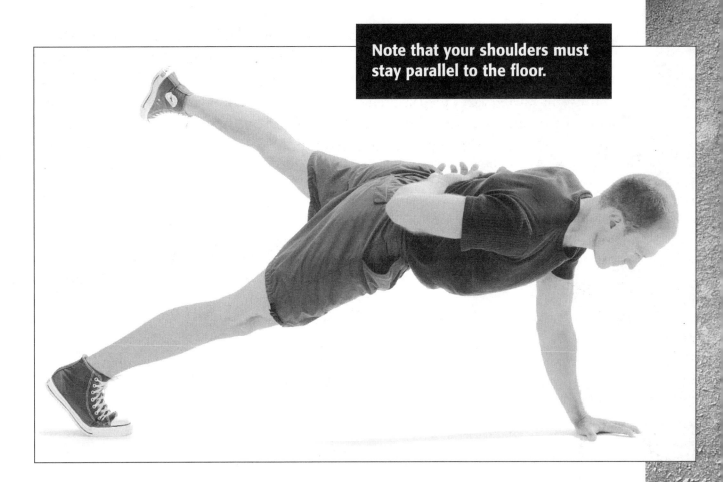

Note that your shoulders must stay parallel to the floor.

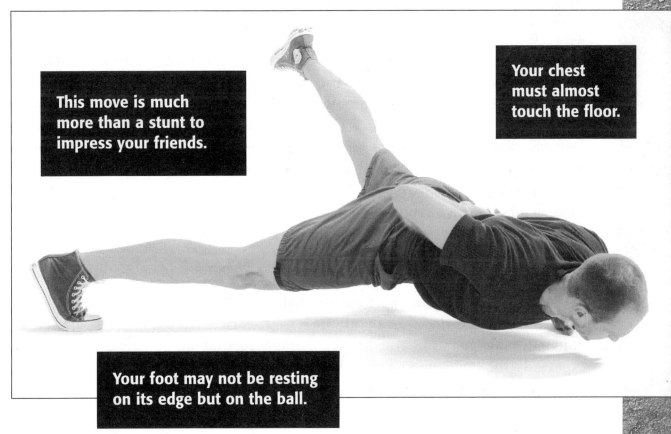

This move is much more than a stunt to impress your friends.

Your chest must almost touch the floor.

Your foot may not be resting on its edge but on the ball.

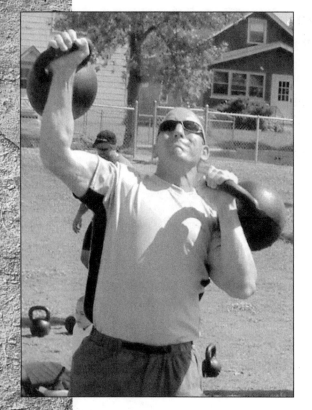

Senior Russian kettlebell instructor Brett Jones has called the one-arm/one-leg pushup "an exercise in total body tension." Photo courtesy Dennis Armstrong, *Dragon Door Publications.*

Brett Jones—RKC Sr., champion of the First Tactical Strength Challenge, owner of InMotionAthletics.com, and all-around strong guy—has called the one-arm/one-leg pushup "an exercise in total body tension." As you will find out when you have finally conquered this challenge, it is impossible to do this exercise without applying all the Naked Warrior performance techniques. Thus, its value goes far beyond strengthening the pushing muscles of the upper body. Expect an awesome midsection workout and a honed skill to tense your muscles for great strength, which can be applied elsewhere.

"One of the most important elements in gymnastics conditioning is body tension or 'body tightness'," writes former gymnast Brad Johnson in one of his exceptional articles on dragondoor.com. "A gymnast can control the action of his or her body more easily, whether in a static strength position or in movement, when his or her body is held tight than when it is a loose collection of individual parts. A person's weight is much more difficult to handle when his or her body is relaxed than if it is held tight. This is why demonstrators at a protest will relax their bodies (go dead weight) when the police are trying to escort or carry them away. By learning and practicing these tension techniques many advanced bodyweight strength movements will become much easier to accomplish."

Good luck finding a muscle that is not working hard during a one-arm/one-leg pushup. Even your lats, unlikely as it may sound, will be working like dogs.

Another advantage of the one-arm pushup is extra shoulder safety. You will not likely overwork your shoulder, as so frequently happens with conventional pushups. You simply cannot do that many one-arm pushups, especially the one-legged variation, even over the course of a day!

But before you can fly, you need to learn how to walk. So follow the very detailed instructions provided later in this book for working up to this awesome move.

GTG is the ultimate specialization program. By definition, you cannot specialize on many things. *The Naked Warrior* will have you do only pistols, and one-arm pushups, period. The warrior is naked and has few weapons. But he uses them expertly.

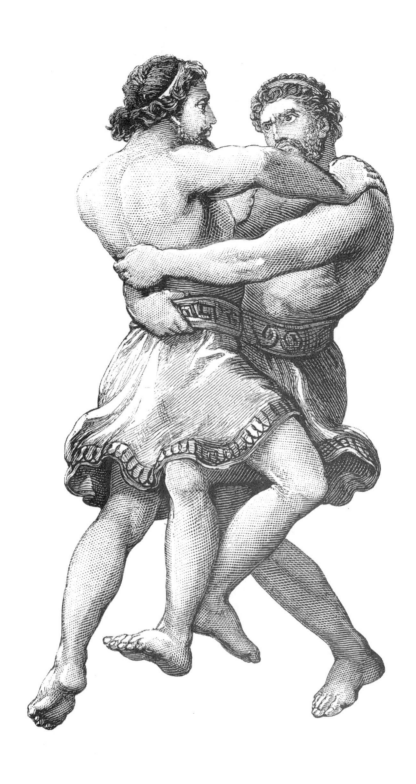

CHAPTER THREE

HIGH-TENSION TECHNIQUES FOR INSTANT STRENGTH

- Tension. What force is made of
- "Raw strength" versus "technique"
- Low gear for brute force
- "Doesn't dynamic tension act like a brake?"
- The power of a fist
- Accidental discharge of strength: A tip from firearms instructors
- Power abs = power body
- Put your "rear-wheel drive" in high gear
- A gymnast instantly gains 40 pounds of strength on his iron cross with the three techniques you have just learned
- The "static stomp": Using ground pressure to maximize power
- Fire your lats and keep your shoulders down: a secret of top karatekas and bench pressers
- "The corkscrew": Another secret of the karate punch

- Bracing: Boost your strength up to 20% with an armwrestling tactic
- "Body hardening"—Tough love for teaching tension
- Beyond bracing: "Zipping up"
- Wind up for power

You have gone over the basics of the Naked Warrior program. Now for the nuts and bolts.

Tension. What force is made of

Spectacular levels of strength can be achieved by increasing the intensity of the muscular contraction.

"Why does correct bodyweight conditioning work so well?" asks gymnastics coach Christopher Sommer. "There are several [reasons], the first is contraction. Basically, the harder the contraction over a greater part of the body during an exercise, the more effective the exercise. For maximum improvement, training to failure is not necessary but maximum contraction is. One of the main advantages to these advanced bodyweight exercises is that they require a complete, full-body contraction. In fact, at advanced levels, they are so demanding that it is simply not possible to complete them any other way."

Tension = Force. The tenser your muscles are, the more strength you will display and build. The Naked Warrior drills will teach you how to get stronger **by contracting your muscles harder.** Expect your strength to start growing from day 1.

Tension = Force.
You can increase your strength
beyond what you thought
possible by contracting your
muscles harder.

Over the centuries, martial artists—as well as gymnasts, lifters, and some other tough hombres—have quietly developed a number of highly effective techniques that greatly enhance strength by channeling the body's scattered energy into the target muscles. These *high-tension techniques (HTTs)* will maximize your strength by forcing your muscles to contract harder. The Naked Warrior program has systematized them into a straightforward method of getting you strong—fast.

Systematic application of the martial arts high-tension techniques (HTTs) will dramatically increase your strength by maximizing muscular tension.

If you are an experienced martial artist, you will likely discover that you are already familiar with many of these techniques. The question is, then, why haven't you been applying them to your strength training? Why don't you teach them? And if you do, why does it take your students years just to start figuring these things out?

I don't claim to have invented these power-generation techniques, but I will take the credit for organizing them into a logical system that can be taught in days, even hours.

"Pavel succinctly explained and applied in a few hours the same principles it took me 10 years to figure out practicing kung-fu" said Jeff Martone, RKC Sr., a defensive tactics and physical training instructor for federal nuclear security teams. Jeff's comment is typical of those I receive after my military and law enforcement courses, which feature the Naked Warrior principles of maximum tension/force generation. Tension is the Naked Warrior's secret weapon.

"Raw strength" versus "technique"

"It's all technique." This is a typical ego saving comment by a bodybuilder who is rubbing his pumped up arm—his butt handed to him on the armwrestling table by a guy with pipes half his size. Sure, and so is the bench press.

It is, in fact! In a recent study, subjects increased their bicep strength 13 percent in three months by simply visualizing tensing their biceps hard but doing no exercise whatsoever. The only possible explanation for this strength gain is greater tension through increased "nerve force".

Let's have world bench press champion George Halbert set things straight: "The most important aspect one can learn to improve strength is to learn proper technique. There is a mode of thinking out there that I describe as 'He's not strong, he's just got good technique.' This is just confused thinking. . . . Have you ever heard anyone say 'He is not a good shooter, he just has good technique' or 'He's not really fast, he just has good technique'?"

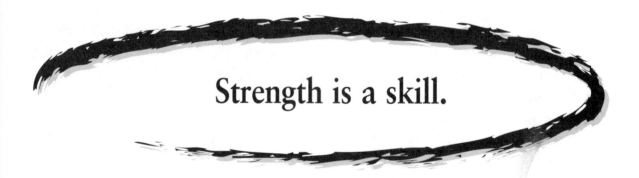

Strength is a skill.

Admiring the performance of "dumb" muscles over focus and honed "nerve force" is just plain dumb. At our booth at the Arnold Schwarzenegger Fitness Expo, we posted a challenge to anyone who could do a strict military press of our 88-pound kettlebell, an awkward monster with a thick, smooth handle. We didn't even require that the bell had to be cleaned to avoid hearing the "This is just technique," bruised ego nonsense. All we wanted was a strict, knees-locked military press.

Strongmen and lifters had no problem putting up the bell, but 220 to 250 bodybuilders failed miserably. On the other hand, our senior Russian Kettlebell Challenge™ instructor Rob Lawrence can press the 88-pounder at 165 pounds of bodyweight and a height of 5 foot, 11 inches. Rob is an example of 'smart muscle'. A wiry karateka, he *practices* his strength rather than *works out*. Another RKC, British kickboxer Nick Fraser, presses the same bell at a bodyweight of 154.

Treat your strength training as a *practice*, rather than a *workout*.

Is it "all technique"? You bet! Does it undermine these gentlemen's accomplishments? No, it elevates them. Are you more humiliated when a big guy kicks your butt or a small one?

In any endeavor, including strength training, mental focus delivers more than physical transformation. Just watch a wiry old karate master chop a pile of bricks in half—a feat that would send a young bodybuilder to the emergency room.

Rob Lawrence, RKC Sr., on the girevoy sport platform. Rob emphasizes exacting technique, mental concentration and the development of wiry strength. Photo courtesy *PhiladelphiaKettlebellClub.net.*

Low gear for brute force

Nine-hundred-pound deadlifter Mark Henry once said, "What makes a good powerlifter is a slow gear." In other words, when you need to pull a car out of the ditch, you call a tow truck, not a Ferrari.

Explosive lifting is the rage these days, and there is no doubt that it's great for many things. Just not for building brute grinding strength. Russian research is clear on this point. [If you want references, ping me on the dragondoor.com forum.]

To anticipate your question, no, such training will not make you slower in your martial arts and sports. The Sanchin kata does not hold back its practitioners, does it? Just understand that few sports are as narrowly focused on max strength as powerlifting. You will have to work on your explosiveness separately. Most sports require you to "drive in multiple gears." This book focuses entirely on "low gear," which gets little or no attention elsewhere.

An emphasis on speed compromises the tension. One of the most crucial skills in the performance of any strength athlete—be it a gymnast, a powerlifter, or an arm wrestler—is the ability to stay tight. "Stay tight!" is the shout you will hear more than any other at any power meet. And only the elite can stay tight while exploding like a bat out of hell. Even the Westside Barbell Club powerlifters, famous for their trademark explosive training, dedicate a special day in their schedule to 'grinding'. So forget pyrotechnics displays until you master full-body tension and your strength starts impressing.

> One of the most crucial strength skills is 'staying tight'. The emphasis on speed compromises the tension.

Rob Lawrence, RKC Sr., made an insightful post on the dragondoor.com forum: "…The trick is to move as quickly as possible without sacrificing the level of tension necessary to sustain the load. If you want to whip your arm out in front of you, it should be as loose as possible; but if you want to push up a bench press, the speed will necessarily be limited by the amount of tension you need to maintain to support the barbell.

"Beginners should emphasize tension first! If you try to teach speed right off the bat, the trainee will confuse 'moving fast' with 'making jerky movements.' Two different things. That is why *Power to the People!* emphasizes tension above all. Once you have the requisite base of tension, that's when you start trying to ramp up the speed. Sometimes someone stuns me by "getting it" (i.e. the mix of speed/tension) the first time they handle weights. The woman who came to my kettlebell class last night, for example, was pressing two 12kg bells with total authority (and speed) in her second KB class. Truly impressive."

Eventually you can speed up—but only if you maintain max tension.

This doesn't mean that you should do the exaggerated 10-second reps that are fashionable (I couldn't have picked a more fitting word) in sissified health clubs, which are also known for pink dumbbells and boy bands. You shouldn't purposefully slow down, just like you shouldn't purposefully speed up. Focus on staying tight as a gymnast. Be cool as Steve McQueen, and the speed will take care of itself.

Don't panic by gunning the rep. You own it. This is the confidence of real strength.

"Doesn't dynamic tension act like a brake?"

The Naked Warrior approach insists that you tense all your muscles when exerting max force. This demand conjures up images of the Okinawan kata Sanchin, in which your own antagonistic muscles provide the resistance.

A natural reaction is: "That tension is going to make me weaker as I am fighting my own muscles, not stronger!"

Wrong. That may be true for dynamic efforts, such as punches and single-joint bodybuilding exercises such as leg curls or leg extensions. But multijoint strength drills, such as one-arm pushups and pistols play by a totally different set of rules.

The agonist/antagonist relationship is pretty straightforward in, say, leg curls or leg extensions. The quads work; the hams impede them. The hams contract; the quads hold them back. Learn to relax the hams, and the quads will get stronger. The proponents of so-called 'muscle control', which was popular at the dawn of weightlifting, tried to do just that. And then there are the compound strength exercises. Take a close look at a squat, barbell, or bodyweight—it makes no difference. Both the quadriceps and the hamstrings are working toward the common goal of standing up. The quads are extending the knees, and the hammies are extending the hips.

A dirty little secret of bodybuilding is that one of the best ways to build the biceps is with the powerlifting-style wide-grip bench press. Your bis may fight your tris in doing skull crushers, but they assist your triceps, deltoids, and pecs in the bench press or the one-arm pushup. In multijoint, high-resistance exercises, the antagonists often act as synergists, especially in experienced athletes. In other words, the "brakes" become "engines."

> In multijoint, high-resistance exercises, the "brakes" become "engines." It is an elite skill that takes time to finesse.

So, the good news is that you can amplify your strength by drawing on the power of the muscles in a way that was traditionally thought to impede their movement. Now, for the bad news: This is an elite skill that takes time to develop and hone. Just like relaxing the antagonist muscles for striking, tensing them properly to enhance your pullup or pushup strength isn't something you master overnight. You might fight yourself a little in the beginning, but this will pass with experience. If it were easy, everybody would be doing it.

As old-timer Maxick wrote in *Great Strength by Muscle Control*, "...when a lifter pulled a barbell" —never mind the barbell, it applies to any type of resistance—"...his mind was concentrated on the barbell or weight and not on the muscles employed. His object was to get the weight aloft; to the muscles that were performing the task he paid no attention. The whole action was therefore controlled to a considerable extent by the weight; consequently a number of available groups of muscles were either left inoperative when they might have been usefully employed, or were brought into play unnecessarily, to the hampering of the lifting muscles."

Mindless lifting is for losers.

The power of a fist

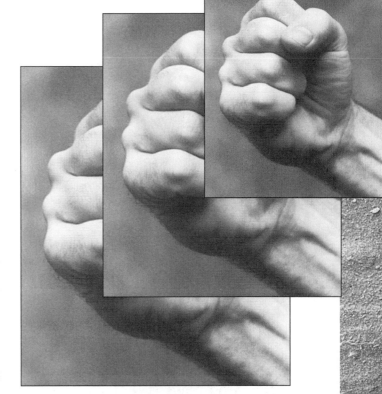

Hit the deck and give me 5 pushups, comrade! Only 5 but of a challenging variety—for instance, with your feet up or on one arm. When you are done with 5, you should be able to grind out another couple but no more than that. Please do pushups on your hands, not your fists, fins, or fingertips. That way, you will do a better job of driving the Naked Warrior principles of power generation home.

Note the difficulty of your first set. Rest briefly. Do another fiver but with one difference: On the way up, grip the deck hard with your fingertips. Don't go up on your fingertips; just grip the floor so that your fingertips turn white. Do this only on the way up. Experiment with whether you get the best results by gripping all the way up or just at the sticking point.

You cannot help noticing that your arms suddenly received a jolt of extra energy, as if your tensing forearms sent some juice up into your triceps. That is exactly what has happened. Whenever a muscle contracts, it irradiates a 'nerve force' around it and increases the intensity of the neighboring muscles' contractions.

Make a fist.

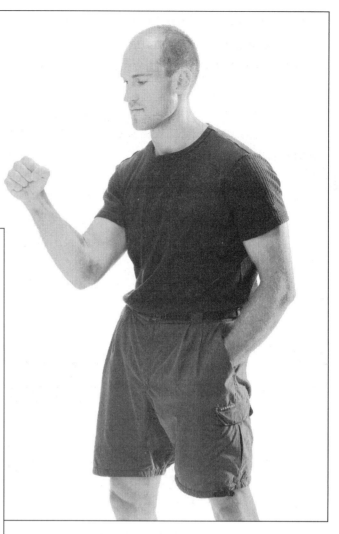

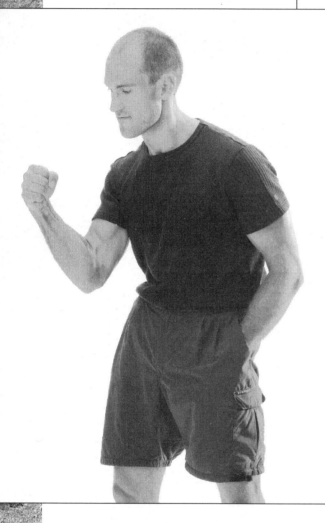

A tight fist. A white-knuckle fist!

Note that as you grip harder, the tension in your forearm overflows into your upper arm and even your shoulder and armpit.

You will increase your strength in any upper body exertion by strongly gripping the floor, the bar, etc. What is truly remarkable is that tightening your fists can enhance your leg strength, as well! Go into a full squat. Pause on the bottom for a second and then get up. Do a couple of reps to take note of the amount of effort it takes you to stand up. On your next squat, make white-knuckle fists at the moment you are about to get up. You will find that doing the squat has become easier! This technique will soon help you tackle the awesome one-legged squat, or pistol.

Your toes can do for your legs what your fingers can do for your arms. Grip the deck with your toes as you are coming out of a squat. You will increase the intensity of the contraction of your hips and power up with ease.

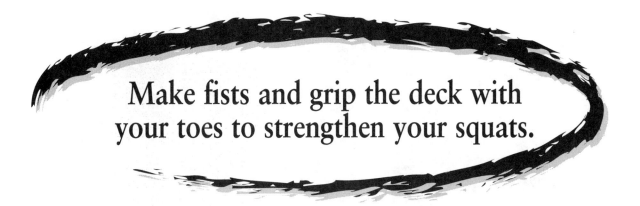

Make fists and grip the deck with your toes to strengthen your squats.

Accidental discharge of strength: A tip from firearms instructors

Your hands are "connected" through "muscle software". One hand imitates the other. A sudden effort with one hand will cause a reflexive contraction of up 20 percent of that intensity in the muscles of the other.

This phenomenon of interlimb response puts fear into the hearts of firearms instructors the world over. They warn against placing your finger on the trigger until you are ready to shoot. If you keep your finger on the trigger, any movement with your other hand—for instance, turning on a flashlight or opening a door—could make your gun go off, due to this squeeze response.

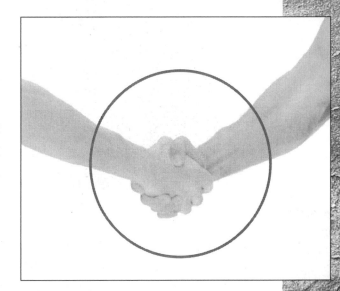

What can land a cop in trouble can help you in your strength training.

Try this test: Squeeze your training partner's hand as hard as possible.

Squeeze your training partner's hand as hard as possible...

...and again, while making a hard fist with your free hand.

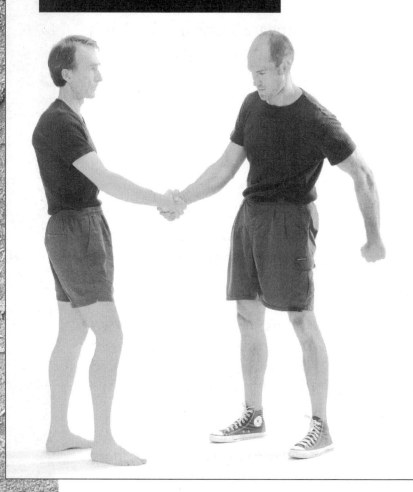

And once more, but this time, also make a hard fist with your free hand.

When you have reached the sticking point in a one-arm strength exercise for the upper body, such as the one-arm pushup, suddenly make a white-knuckle fist or tightly grip the surface or bar with your free hand. Doing so will fire up your strength and get you unstuck.

In one-arm upper body exercises, fire the gripping muscles of your free hand at the sticking point.

This strategy works well in the context of many punches in karate and other hard styles. The instant your reverse punch nails the target, make a hard fist with your nonstriking hand. You cannot help but notice the "power line" that connects your fists.

Power abs = A power body

"All my attention, all my training, all my thinking is centered on my abdomen."
—Mas Oyama

Tensing your abs will amplify the intensity of the contraction of any muscle in your body.

Martial arts masters have instinctively understood this phenomenon for centuries, and you are about experience it yourself. But don't rush to hit the deck and apply it to pushups. Chances are, you don't even know how to contract your abs properly.

The "crunch generation" has been brainwashed into sucking in their waspy waists when working their abs. Big sissies. You are supposed to have your core tight and full of compressed energy. You are supposed to feel anchored in your lower abdomen. What do you feel in your belly when you suck it in? Like a weak, disconnected beauty queen. Go get a manicure.

You need to understand several things. First, a muscle contracts in a straight line, not in a curve. So your abs should draw your sternum and pubic bone together in a straight line, not a semicircle. Second, for boring, geeky reasons that I will leave out, when you suck in your stomach, your intra-abdominal pressure (or 'Ki' or 'Chi', if you insist) drops off. The bottom line is this: Flat abs are strong abs.

Flat abs are strong abs; a sucked in stomach is weak.

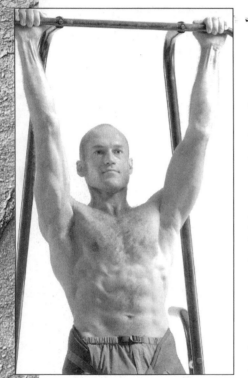

You will not get stronger until you learn to contract your abdominals flat and strong. Doing the following 'back-pressure crunch' will teach you how. Assume the regular crunch position, your knees at 90 degrees and your feet flat on the floor. Now, instead of focusing on crunching up, **put all your effort into pressing your lower back down hard.** I picked up this tip from Aussie author Kit Laughlin, and it's so good that it almost makes the crunch a worthwhile exercise in its own right.

When you press down on the area of your back that would be covered by a karate belt, a few cool things will happen. Your spine will naturally round. Both your trunk and your pelvis will come up just like the ends of a mattress curl when a big guy flops in the middle, and you will be unable to come up any higher than you are supposed to in doing a crunch. You just cannot sit up when your lower back is grounded.

This unusual maneuver is out of the jurisdiction of your hip flexors, which means more work for your dear abbies. Finally, the back-pressure crunch will make your abs contract in a straight line, as they are supposed to.

The back-pressure crunch works even better if you stick something like a rolled-up yoga mat under your back. You will work your abs through a longer range of motion, and you will find it easier to press down.

To sum up, don't worry about crunching, rolling up, or sitting up. Just focus on pressing your lower back into the deck as hard as possible. Place your hands on your abs as you are crunching and note the sensation; you are supposed to be able to reproduce it in any context. Once you can, try the following strength test.

Shake hands with a partner, both of you squeezing as hard as possible. Have him note how hard your grip is. Rest briefly and repeat the test, your partner doing nothing different and you adding the ab flex into the mix.

Keep your abdominals short and flat; reproduce the sensation you experience while doing back-pressure crunches. One more time: When flexing your stomach, do not suck it in or stick it out. Brace it as you would for a punch (that can be arranged). You (or rather your sparring partner) will notice your greater hand strength.

Power to you!

Keep your abdominals short and flat.

When flexing your stomach, do not suck it in or stick it out.

Brace it as you would for a punch.

Put your "rear-wheel drive" in high gear

Experienced fighters are not impressed with large pipes. They know that real striking power is generated in the hips. One karate master even stated that makiwara punching is meant to strengthen the hips, rather than the knuckles. Boxing coach Steve Baccari, RKC, told me that Mike Tyson's arms measure 16 inches in diameter and that Evander Holyfield's are 15. Either would be large on a 160-pound, 5-feet, five-inch bodybuilder, but you have to agree that these numbers seem pretty average for a heavyweight.

Yet most people, even athletes, are preoccupied with their arms and don't have a clue how to recruit their glutes, the strongest muscles in their bodies. You must acquire this skill because no strength exercise or martial arts technique will be effective without your knowing how to create high tension in your hip muscles. Tom Furman, RKC, aptly referred to these all-important muscles as the "rear-wheel drive."

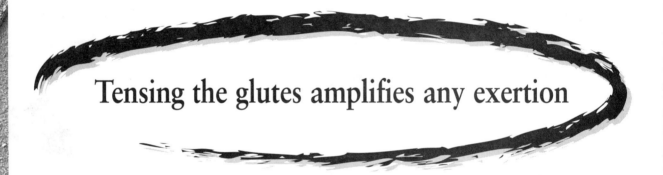

Tensing the glutes amplifies any exertion

An effective image is **pinching a coin with your cheeks**. Silly but effective.

Back to our handgrip test. In addition to the contracting your abs, lock your glutes as you are crushing your friend's hand. You will be stronger. I guarantee it.

A gymnast instantly gains 40 pounds of strength on his iron cross with the three techniques you have just learned

From *The Power of Tension*, by Brad Johnson. © 2002 by Brad Johnson. Reprinted by permission.

I recently reported the results of a crude experiment on the effects of tension techniques on strength performance. Since Pavel asked me to write an article, I decided to repeat the experiment with a better design and more precise measurements.

The strength exercise that I used was the Iron Cross. I stood on a bathroom scale while pushing down on the rings to measure the amount of my own bodyweight that I could lift off the scale with a variety of tension conditions. I rested my hands on the rings and extended my locked arms to an angle approximately 20 degrees above the perfect Iron Cross position (a slight Y instead of a T shape). This angle increased the leverage disadvantage of the exercise and I was fairly certain that I would not be able to lift my body completely off the scale. I used four tension conditions:

(1) pushing down on the rings as hard as I could without any of the following three tension techniques,
(2) squeezing the rings as hard as I could,
(3) tensing my abdominal muscles,
(4) tensing my glutes.

I repeated all four of these conditions six times. I always started with condition number one and then varied the order of the remaining three conditions. For example, the first sequence was 1, 2, 3, 4 and the second sequence was 1, 3, 4, 2. Each sequence, I would add one tension technique at a time so that I could measure their cumulative effects. On the first sequence I measured strength:

(1) with no tension technique,
(2) with hand squeeze,
(3) with hand squeeze + ab squeeze,
(4) with hand squeeze + ab squeeze + glute squeeze.

All sequences were done in that manner. I decided to measure six sequences so that I performed each possible order of the three tension techniques. This allowed me to calculate the individual as well as the cumulative strength contributions of the three tension techniques and gave me more data to visually examine for patterns.

In each condition, I pressed down on the rings as hard as I could. I attempted to utilize only the prescribed tension technique(s). This was challenging because I was accustomed to utilizing all of them together. I pressed down for approximately three seconds and watched the needle on the scale. Although the needle was shaking (a range of 4 to 6 pounds), it was pretty easy to find the center point. I recorded the weight and rested for one minute before the next condition. I observed my scores on the first and last condition of each sequence to make sure that my performance was not affected by fatigue. These scores were almost identical throughout the experiment.

Now for the good stuff! The average strength increase from the use of the 3 tension techniques combined was 40.33 pounds. The average cumulative strength increases for the separate conditions were: hand squeeze—8.5 pounds, ab squeeze—20.33 pounds, and glute squeeze—11.17 pounds. There were two sequences where each of the tension techniques was the first and, therefore, the only one used. The average strength increase for each condition when it was the only technique utilized was: hand squeeze—10 pounds, ab squeeze—30 pounds, and glute squeeze—13.5 pounds.

In conclusion, I knew that the tension techniques increased strength but I was surprised by the size of the increase. I imagine that the strength increases of the individual and combined tension techniques vary depending upon the selected exercise and the athlete. I realize that I committed all kinds of experimental errors but the results were more than enough to convince me of the POWER OF TENSION!!!

I hope that this report of the experiment was clear. If not, I would be glad to answer any questions about it on the dragondoor.com forum.

Comrade, pay attention to every performance tip in this book!
Read, practice, then read and practice some more. The fine points
of power generation are much more important than the
individual exercises. If you skip the High Tension Techniques and go
directly to the cals you are not practicing the Naked Warrior
moves but wasting your time. If you have attention deficit
disorder, you have no business strength training.

The "static stomp":
Using ground pressure to maximize power

Karate great Masatoshi Nakayama used to say, "Motive power comes from the powerful thrust of the supporting leg; the principle is the same as that of the jet engine. . . . The vital core of the movement is the reaction between the supporting leg and the floor. The greater this reaction is, the faster the body advances."

Focus on applying maximum pressure to the deck with your foot when doing the pistol and with your palm when doing the one-arm pushup. Push straight though the platform, as Olympic weightlifters like to say. Imagine that you are stomping down. Yes, a "static stomp!" For a number of reasons—physical, psychological, and physiological—doing so will translate into a more powerful contraction of your pushing muscles.

Go ahead. Stand on one foot and press it harder and harder into the deck. Assume the top position of the one-arm pushup and do the same with your hand. Feel the steady build-up of tension? If you try the same from the bottom, you will spring right up.

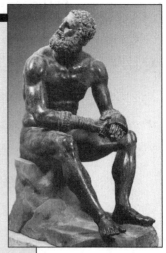

APPLY MAX PRESSURE TO THE FLOOR WITH YOUR PALM OR FOOT. PUSH STRAIGHT THROUGH THE DECK. STRIVE FOR THE SENSATION OF MAXIMUM PRESSURE WITH "A STATIC STOMP".

"Stomp" with the whole surface of your palm or the sole of your foot with the emphasis on the heel. The heel of the foot and the heel of the palm. The heel of the palm is the spot at the base of the palm below the little finger. It is the spot used in palm strikes. Applying pressure to this spot structurally aligns the arm to be very strong and fires up the triceps and lat.

In one-arm pushups also keep your legs rigid and push the balls of your feet through the floor. Everything in your body is interrelated and isolation is a myth. Try it; it works.

Everything in your body is interrelated and isolation is a myth.

Downstairs, the heel pressure will recruit your powerful rear-wheel drive. The application does not have to be static; weightlifters use it during jerks for instance. "I always stomp a few hard ones with each foot before a heavy squat, and can always grind out a few more pounds as the result," says Dan 'Garm' Bescher, RKC, whose tough guy record includes combat with the Recon Marines, a world drug free powerlifting title, and an impressive martial arts background. "I try to hit with a flat foot, and really send a shock wave back up the leg. This is a common technique in Xinyiquan kung fu."

Tense your lats and keep your shoulders down: a secret of top karatekas and bench pressers

Shrugging your shoulder and/or letting it move forward will destroy your shoulder and your power alike—whether you are punching, benching, or doing pushups. You are in effect 'disconnecting' your arm from your powerful torso muscles.

Masatoshi Nakayama used to say, "The shoulders must always be kept low. . . . If the shoulders rise, . . . the muscles in the side of the body will soften, and power cannot be concentrated." The master was speaking about the punch, but the one-arm pushup is no different. "Hips, chest, shoulder, arm, wrist and fist—all must be firmly linked together, and all muscles must function fully. But if the shoulder is raised when punching, or leads the movement of the body, the muscles around the armpit will not contract properly, no matter how much arm muscles are contracted. Then the impact will probably cause the fist to rebound from the target."

Shrugging your shoulder or moving it forward is 'disconnecting' your arm from your powerful torso muscles.

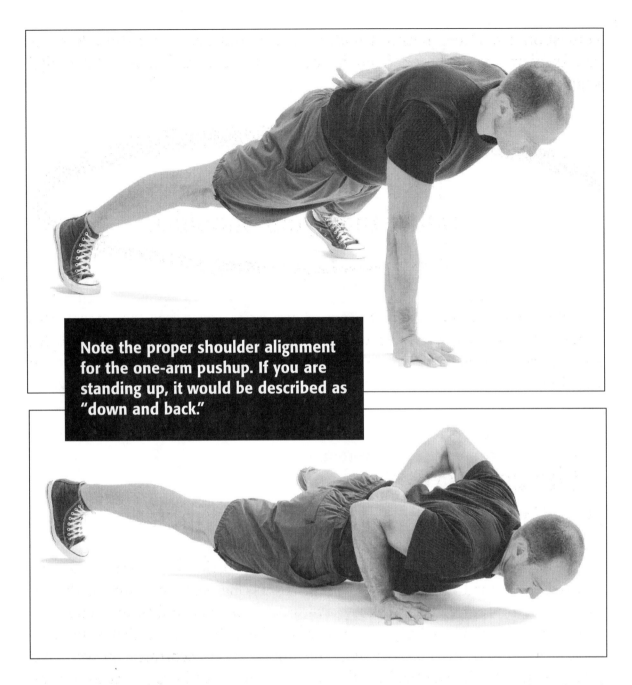

Note the proper shoulder alignment for the one-arm pushup. If you are standing up, it would be described as "down and back."

Many top powerlifters keep their shoulder pressed down into the bench and toward their feet. As a result, they put up heavier poundages and suffer fewer shoulder injuries. This is no different when you are pushing your bodyweight.

Although it seems natural to keep your energy on the top of your shoulder and to push with it, doing so is a recipe for weakness and injury. "Throughout the punch [and the one-arm pushup], minimize tension on the outside of the arm and over the shoulder to maintain a smooth arch [of energy transmission]—tensing the latissimus dorsi and serratus anterior muscles (along the ribs)—to transfer stress," insists Lester Ingber, doctor of physics and karate sensei. In other words, push from your armpit, rather than your shoulder. "Keep tensions under the arm and avoid stiff shoulders that can disconnect the block from it source of speed and mass, the body," suggests Ingber.

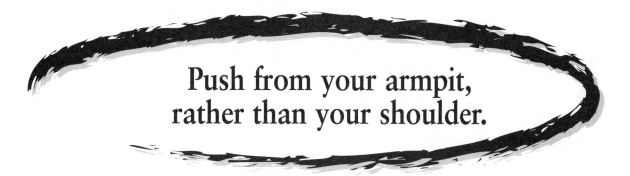

Push from your armpit, rather than your shoulder.

While it may seem counterintuitive to you right now, once you master this concept of armpit power, you will wonder how you ever did without it. It's going to pay off big in your one-arm pushups, punches, and bench presses, if you do them.

"The corkscrew": Another secret of the karate punch

"The twisting motion [of a karate punch] contributes to setting a true course," explained the late Nakayama. "The principle is the same as that of rifling in a gun barrel. Without the rifling, the bullet would tumble end over end and veer from its course. Because of the rifling, the bullet spins and travels a true course... Twisting the forearm concentrates power and amplifies it. This is true because the twisting causes an instantaneous tensing of all the muscles involved in the technique."

A threaded firearm is superior to a flat-barreled one.

Rotation, or spiral tension, increases the stability and power of almost any action.

This is the essence of the corkscrew principle. Gripping the rifle while isometrically twisting both hands in opposite directions—the right clockwise and the left counterclockwise—made a dramatic difference for bayonet fighting in the U.S. Marine Corps Martial Arts Program. The Marines' thrusts became more powerful and much harder to deflect. The same is true for strength exercises. Following is a sequence of drills to teach you how it's done.

Hold a stick in front of you, as you would hold a bar for the bench press.

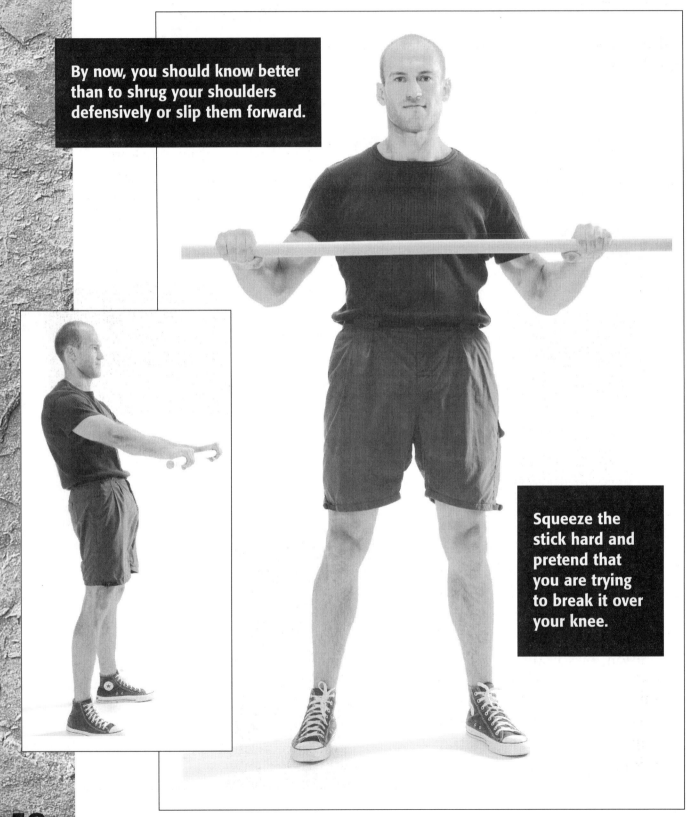

By now, you should know better than to shrug your shoulders defensively or slip them forward.

Squeeze the stick hard and pretend that you are trying to break it over your knee.

You should feel tension in your armpits, your lats, and your pecs. Your elbows will move somewhat in toward your body, and your shoulders will move away from your ears. Top bench pressers flare their lats to drive the bar off their chest. The corkscrew technique is a shortcut to mastering this difficult skill.

If no stick is available, hold your arms in front of you and twist them from inside out as far as possible.

Imagine that you are screwing your arms into your shoulder sockets. You should feel tension from your armpits spiraling toward your fists.

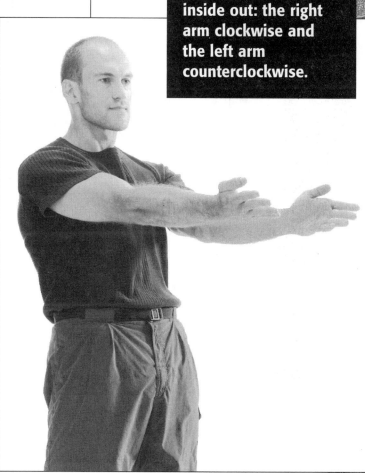

Corkscrew from the inside out: the right arm clockwise and the left arm counterclockwise.

Note that where a karate punch twists from the outside in, a pushup (or a bench press or a palm strike) twists from the inside out. That is, the right arm moves clockwise and the left arm moves counterclockwise. Your shoulders will retract into their sockets and perform more strongly with this external rotation.

Test the corkscrew power in repeating the handshake test.

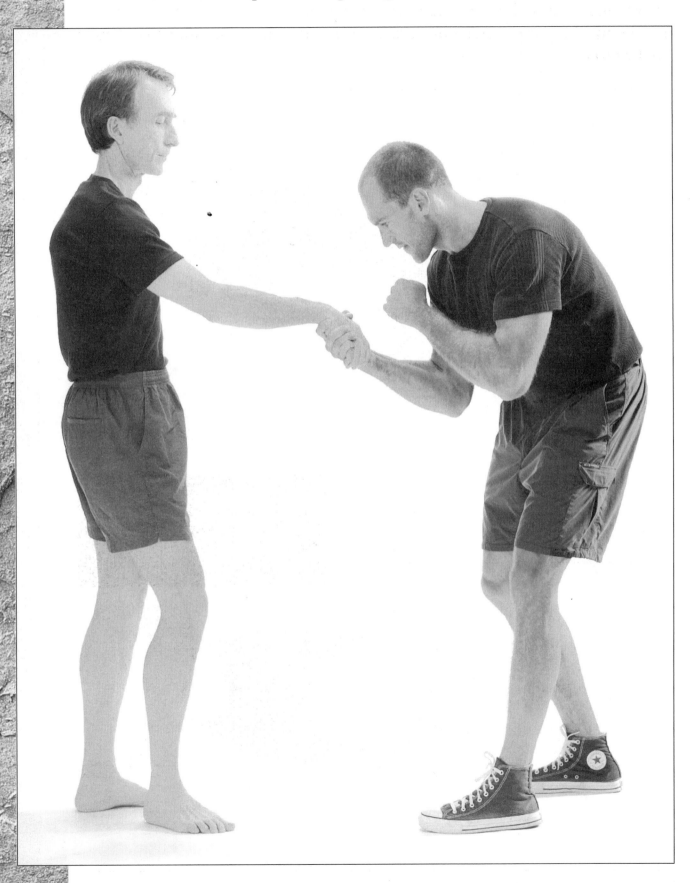

Then hit the deck and give me a couple of regular two-arm pushups. Grip the ground hard with your fingertips, making sure that your hands stay put, and apply the same inside-out corkscrew tension to the ground that you applied to the stick.

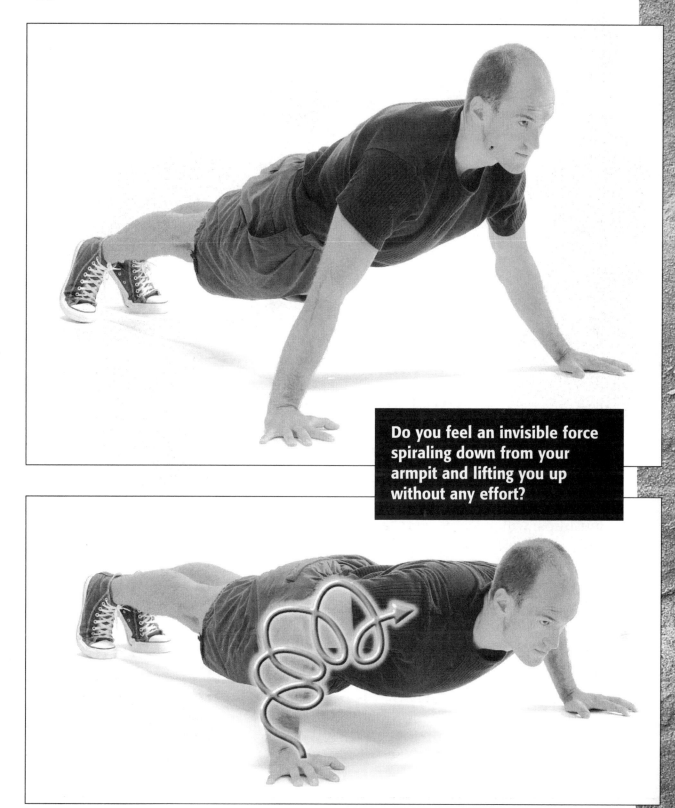

Do you feel an invisible force spiraling down from your armpit and lifting you up without any effort?

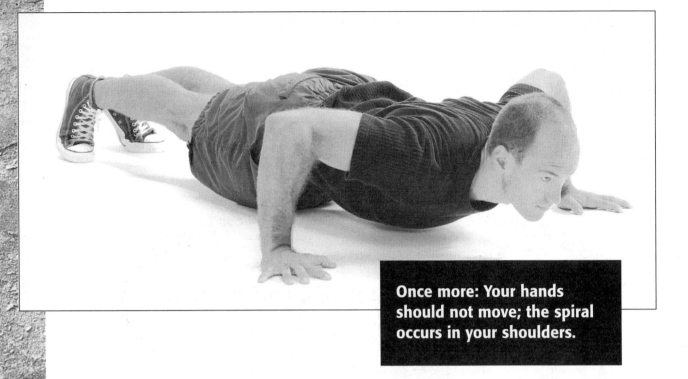

Once more: Your hands should not move; the spiral occurs in your shoulders.

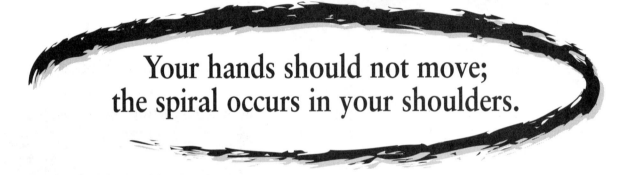

Your hands should not move;
the spiral occurs in your shoulders.

Your fingers should grip the deck hard, but keep your hands stationary. The pushups will become very easy. Your body should feel like it's rising on springs. You should feel a distinct spiral of 'energy' moving from your armpits to your hands.

Bracing: Boost your strength up to 20% with an armwrestling tactic

A decent armwrestler loads all his muscles with high-strung tension before the ref yells 'Go!' A top armwrestler will load even before he grips up with his or her opponent. And an amateur who waits for the referee's command to pull before turning on his biceps finds himself pinned without knowing what has hit him.

According to the father of plyometrics, Russian sports scientist Yuri Verkhoshansky, isometrically tensing your muscles before a dynamic contraction can improve your performance by up to 20 percent. You are about to experience what that means.

> **Pre-tensing your muscles before starting to move can improve your performance by up to 20 percent.**

Do 5 hard pushups, totally relaxing on the deck between reps. Notice how you have to tense up somewhat before pushing up each time? Do another 5, this time making a point of maximally tensing your whole body before pushing up. You should find that you have much more strength.

Attempt a one-arm pushup or another challenging pushup from the position of lying relaxed on the deck. Most likely, you will fail. Now brace your whole body before starting the pushup and successfully complete the attempt.

Loading tension into the muscles before an exertion increases their power. You must learn to brace against resistance the same way you brace against a strike.

The key is to brace yourself before the resistance is upon you; otherwise, it will be too late. Houdini could take anyone's punch if he was prepared for it. He died when he got struck without warning.

Dead-start exercises, such as the one just described, are great for teaching yourself higher tension, especially in your weak links. Because they eliminate the helpful bounce, dead starts greatly challenge the muscles and strengthen them for normal pushups and the like.

So, be sure to include plenty of dead starts in your regimen, once you are strong enough to do them. To do a one-arm pushup, relax completely while lying down on the floor; then tense up and go. Relax at the bottom of a pistol before powering back up. Enjoy the pain!

"Body hardening"— Tough love for teaching tension

Here is how to acquire the bracing skill the quick and hard way.

The U.S. Marine Corps Martial Arts Program has been practicing "body hardening", or controlled striking of fleshy parts of the body to accustom the Marines' bodies to the rigors of contact fighting. The Soviet Spetsnaz did the same thing. You can occasionally see on American television footage of Russian commandos breaking incoming two-by-fours by flexing their traps and taking full-force kicks in the gut. We also applied such drills to teach the body the tightness necessary to lift heavy and safe.

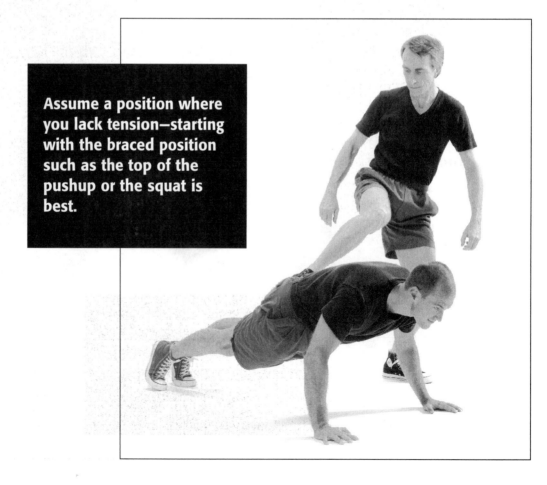

Assume a position where you lack tension—starting with the braced position such as the top of the pushup or the squat is best.

Have a partner pound your muscles with his fists, the ridges of his hands, and his feet. It is not a bad idea to start with the regular two-arm pushup. These strikes should not be of the knockout variety. They shouldn't even hurt or leave bruises if you tighten up on impact. It goes without saying that you should not hit the spine, the bones, the head, and other vulnerable areas.

Your partner should work over your whole musculature—from your calves to your neck. He should give special emphasis to the muscles that you have a real hard time flexing. For instance, if you have a hard time standing upright on one leg because your hip abductors, the muscles outside the thigh, are not firing, then a few careful kicks to the outside of the butt cheek—not to the bony part of the leg—should take care of it.

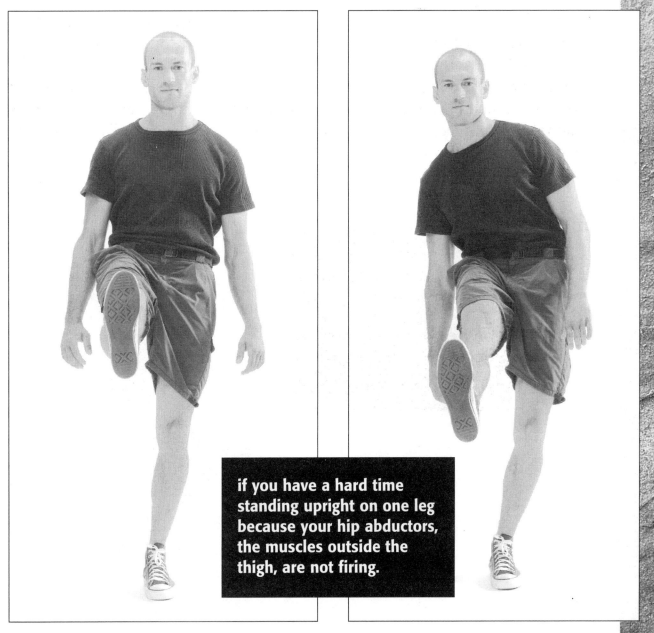

if you have a hard time standing upright on one leg because your hip abductors, the muscles outside the thigh, are not firing.

In the one-arm pushup, the area that needs extra attention is the armpit (that is, the pecs and the lats) and the abs.

In the one-legged squat variation, the obliques, the glutes, and all the muscles around the thigh should get some tough love.

So, get a buddy to give you this treatment—he will be delighted—and you will have this tension thing figured out in no time flat.

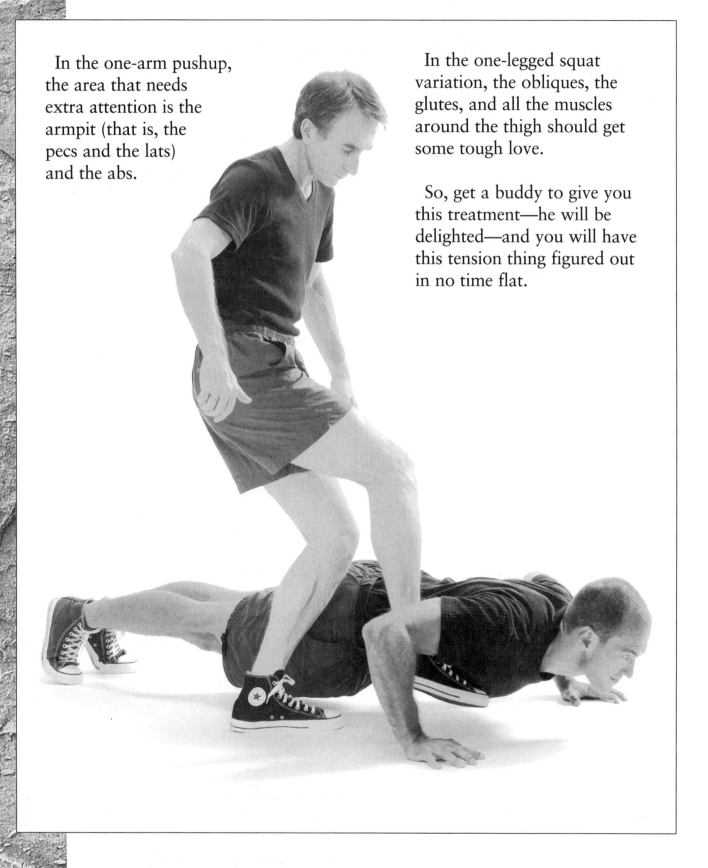

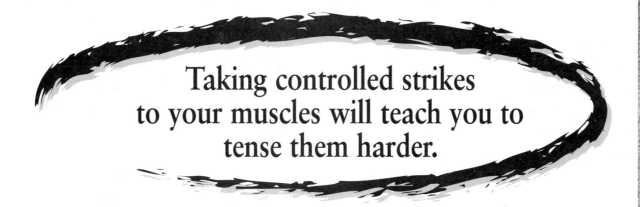

Taking controlled strikes
to your muscles will teach you to
tense them harder.

Beyond bracing: "Zipping up"

A state-of-the-art form of bracing, called "zipping up," will take your pretensing skills to a new level. This technique is somewhat advanced, as it requires good body awareness. If you don't get it at first, revisit it in a few months.

Practice the technique in the braced position: at the top of a one-arm pushup or one-legged squat.

Pull up your kneecaps by tensing your quads. Now focus on pulling your quad up even higher into your groin, as you would window shutters.

Next do the same with the rest of your thigh muscles: the inner, the outer, and the hamstrings. It is as if you have grabbed your leg with both hands just above the knee, squeezed, and slowly **pulled all the thigh muscles up into the groin.** Imagine that you are pulling your thigh up into the hip socket as well.

Try to get that feeling of "zipping up" your muscles; it is very powerful. Your thigh muscles will feel very short, hard, and *retracted* into the hip joint.

Flex your glutes by 'pinching a coin' with your cheeks.

Work up your body. The waist. **Shorten the muscles surrounding your waist—the abs, the obliques, the muscles around your ribs—remembering to keep them flat.** If you have done it right your lower ribs will move in and your stomach will stay flat rather than suck in. Just **zip all your torso muscles from your ribs down to your pelvis.** Breathe shallow as your respiratory muscles get constricted; do not hold your breath.

Up until now the instructions applied to both the pushups and the squats. The following is just for the pushups.

The pecs and lats. Flex them so they pull your shoulders down, away from your ears. B.K.S. Iyengar, a master of Yoga, says, "the traps belong to the back, not the neck." Then **shorten your armpit muscles even further so they pull your shoulders into your body.**

Pull your rigid arms into the shoulder sockets; retract them.

If you can figure out how, **"screw your shoulders into their sockets" from inside out, right arm clockwise, left one counterclockwise.**

Make the biceps and the triceps retreat into the deltoids. It is the same "rolling up of the shades" that you did with your thigh muscles.

Your forearms. **"Gather up" your forearm muscles by your elbows, pull up your forearm bones into the elbows.**

ZIP! You have achieved a very compact and powerful alignment. And if you have not—keep practicing.

The fine points, annoying as they seem, are the meat of the program and the only legit shortcut to strength.

As you get proficient, try zipping up in your dead start drills.

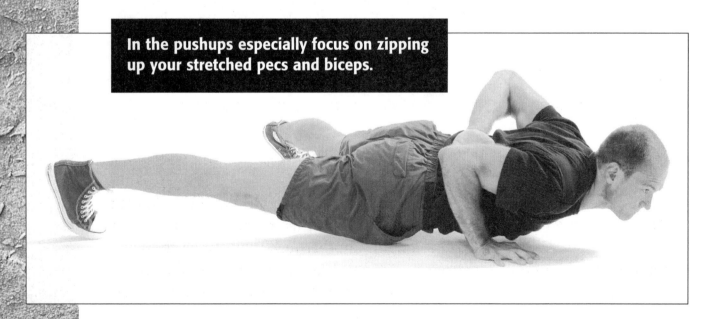

In the pushups especially focus on zipping up your stretched pecs and biceps.

It is harder to zip up a stretched muscle, but if it were easy everyone would be doing it.

In the pushups especially focus on zipping up your stretched pecs and biceps. Push up. You will pop up like a spring.

Work up to practicing zipping up in dead start exercises but don't stop practicing at the lockout.

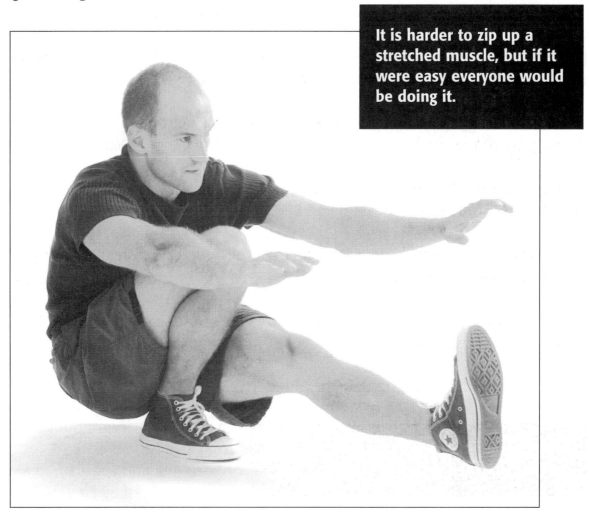

It is harder to zip up a stretched muscle, but if it were easy everyone would be doing it.

Wind up for power

Throw a series of karate punches, and observe how your body gets loaded for each successive punch. "Energy (compression) from compressed muscles can be reused to produce the beginning of another technique much the same as motion can be obtained from a compressed spring or sponge-ball," states Lester Ingber, Ph.D., in his excellent book *Karate Kinematics and Dynamics*.

Strength training is no different. Once you have zipped up your muscles, it should be obvious that you have stored a tremendous amount of elastic energy. You will find it interesting that it can be reused even without a bounce. Here's how.

Instead of going down by yielding to the gravity, actively pull yourself down while still staying braced and tight. In the pushup, pull with your lats and other back muscles; don't forget the inside-out corkscrew on the way down. In the squat, pull with your hip flexors, the muscles on the tops of your thighs whose job it is to jackknife your body. Your zipped-up muscles should feel like stretched rubber bands.

> **Instead of yielding to the gravity, actively pull yourself down while still tight. Imagine that you are stretching your muscles like rubber bands.**

Armed forces powerlifting champion Jack Reape suggests an excellent drill to teach you how to pull yourself into the squat on the dragondoor.com forum: "the reverse squat". "Hold a pulldown rope around the back of your neck, then squat down and bend over. Good for your abs and great for your stabilizers." It will work just as well with a bungee cord hooked to a pullup bar and the one-legged squat.

To drive the active negative concept home for the pushup, try the towel row explained in Chapter 8, the Q&A or a "reverse pushup" pullup. Lie on your back underneath a securely anchored bar, and grab the bar with a palms-over, shoulder-width grip. Make your body rigid and pull your chest to the bar; your feet should stay on the deck. Force your chest out and pull it toward the bar in a rowing motion. Notice what it feels like and try to recreate the same pulling sensation when you are lowering your body for a pushup. Pay attention to stretching your pecs; it will help your rebound big time.

"Internal martial artists figured out how to 'load tension' into their muscles by deliberately twisting their bodies like coiled springs," explains John Du Cane, RKC, in his online Qigong Secrets newsletter, available at dragondoor.com. "This coiled position is either held for long periods or used as a preparation or transition for explosive action. Iron Shirt qigong uses this technique, as do forms like The 18 Buddha Hands and The Five Animal Frolics." The Naked Warrior strength secrets have been out there all along.

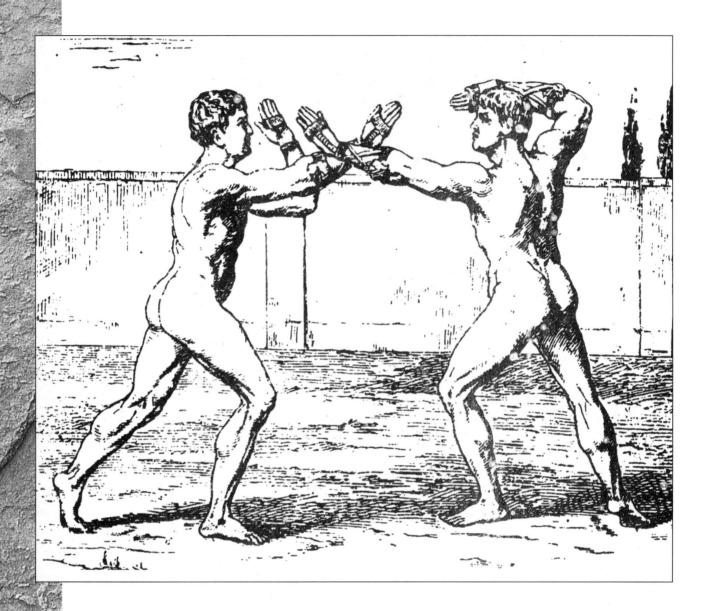

CHAPTER FOUR

POWER BREATHING: THE MARTIAL ARTS MASTERS' SECRET FOR SUPERSTRENGTH

- Bruce Lee called it "breath strength"
- Power inhalation
- "Compression, not exhalation": a Tai Chi master demystifies Power Breathing
- Reverse power breathing: Evolution of the Iron Shirt technique
- Power up from the core, or the "pneumatics of Chi"

⚠ WARNING!

Pressurized breathing is dangerous to persons with high blood pressure, heart problems, or other health concerns! Don't start practicing it without consulting your doctor first.

Bruce Lee called it "breath strength"

The lungs are reservoirs of air, and the air is the lord of strength.
Whoever speaks of strength must know of air.
—Jui Meng, a Shaolin monk, 1692

Bruce Lee used to say that the martial arts rely more on "breath strength" than "body strength." Indeed, cranking up the breath strength will boost the body strength. The effect of breathing patterns and intraabdominal pressure (IAP) on strength is oddly ignored by most Western strength-training authorities. Yet compressed or power breathing is one of the most powerful ways of increasing muscular strength in existence!

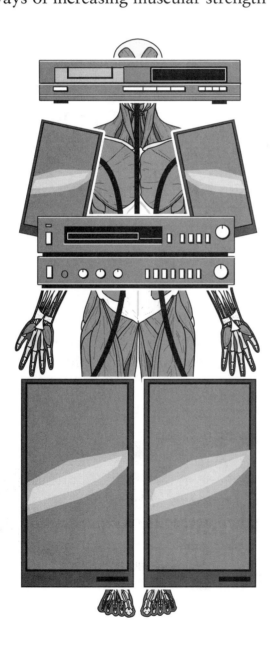

Think of your brain as a CD player. Think of your muscles as the speakers. Where do you think the amplifier is? In your stomach. Special receptors measure the intraabdominal pressure and act as the "volume control knob." When the IAP bottoms out, the tension in all your muscles drops off. In my stretching book, I explain how to take advantage of this phenomenon and make dramatic gains in flexibility overnight.

On the other hand, when the internal pressure goes up, your nervous system gets more excited and the nerve cells supplying your muscles become superconductors of the commands from your brain. So, by cranking up the IAP volume knob, you will automatically get noticeably stronger —in every muscle in your body and with any exercise!

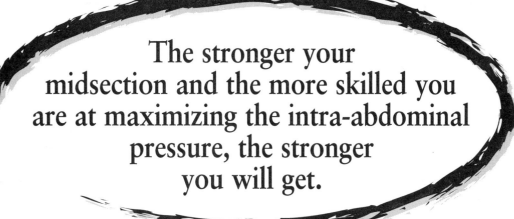

The stronger your midsection and the more skilled you are at maximizing the intra-abdominal pressure, the stronger you will get.

If you have a heart condition, high blood pressure, a hernia or some other health problem you must ask for a specific breathing advice from your doctor. If you are healthy enough to handle it, power breathing will be the best thing that has happened to your strength. Ever.

To make sure we are clear on the definition, **power breathing is a type of breathing that maximizes the intra-abdominal pressure in order to amplify your strength.**

Power inhalation

Note that the operative word here is intra-abdominal—not intra-thoracic. You have nothing good to gain from pressure in your head or chest. Send it down to your stomach!

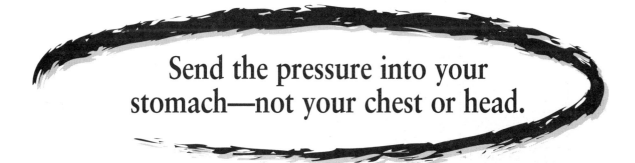

Send the pressure into your stomach—not your chest or head.

Abdominal breathing is a skill that consistently eludes most Western men, especially the ones who puff up with virtual lats and lose the energy in their abdomen.

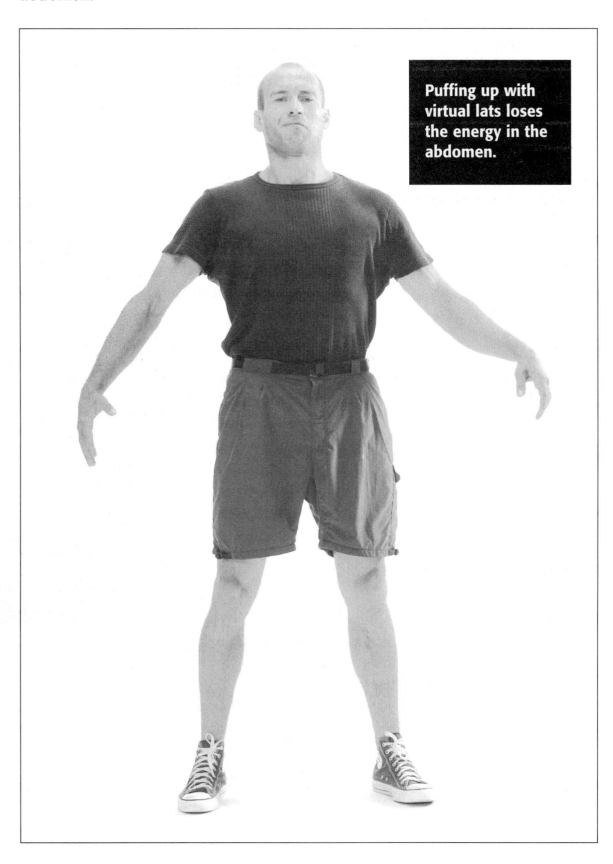

Puffing up with virtual lats loses the energy in the abdomen.

You must override your ego. Let your shoulders deflate, and move your breath and energy down to your abdomen.

This doesn't mean slouching, though. Keep your neck tall and your spine straight.

Drop your shoulders. This drill will help: stand straight, your arms hanging by your sides. Without bending over **reach down as low as possible with your fingertips. Tense your armpits to push your shoulders down away from your ears.** Relax. Your shoulders should stay down better now.

Now imagine that your head is tied to a string and the string is pulling it up. "...stretch your neck up, not forward," stressed Mas Oyama; **without shrugging the shoulders.**

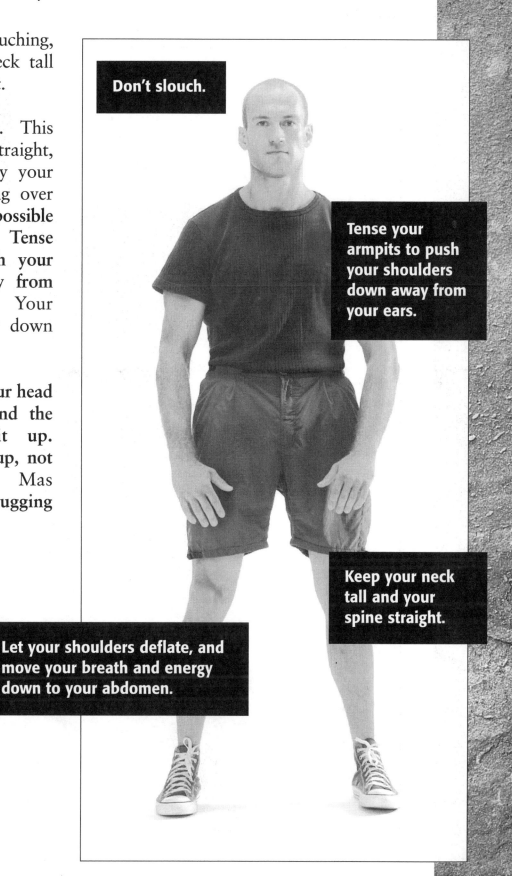

Don't slouch.

Tense your armpits to push your shoulders down away from your ears.

Keep your neck tall and your spine straight.

Let your shoulders deflate, and move your breath and energy down to your abdomen.

Here's another drill: Remove your shoes and lie down on the deck on your back.

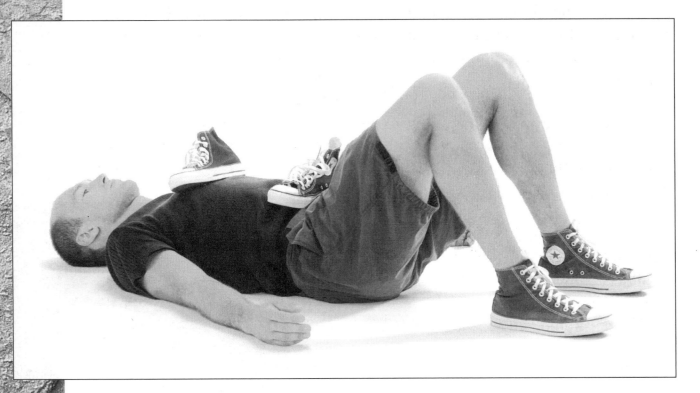

Place one shoe on your stomach and another on your chest. (A barbell plate, a kettlebell, or your training partner sitting down are other viable options.) Practice abdominal breathing through your nose until only the shoe on your belly moves up and down (but the one on your chest does not). Remember this feeling.

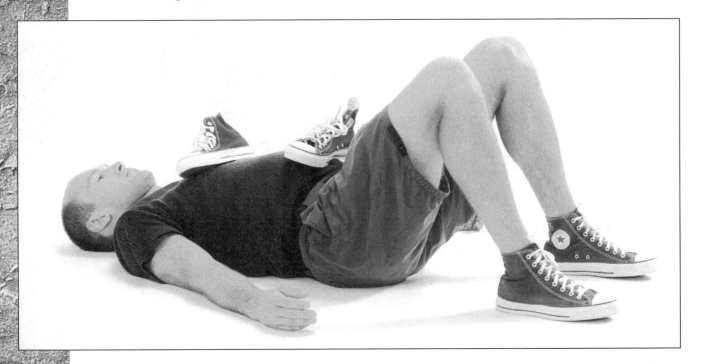

What is abdominal breathing? Technically, you will not be sucking air into your belly because your lungs are upstairs. But your lungs can be expanded by using different sets of muscles. You can inhale by shrugging your shoulders, which is no good. You can inhale by expanding your rib cage, which is better but still doesn't get you a cigar. Or you can inhale by expanding your belly.

Pay attention now. You are about to be introduced to a muscle that is vital to great strength yet never mentioned in bodybuilding magazines or even books on strength training. Perhaps because it is invisible and you can't impress girls with it.

This mystery muscle is the diaphragm. This parachute-shaped contraption separates your lungs from your guts. When your diaphragm contracts, it pushes down and two things happen. First, your lungs get pulled down, too, which creates low pressure in them. Fresh air therefore gets sucked in. Second, your inner organs get pushed down and displaced (unless your abs are tight). Your belly expands. So, stomach breathing is really diaphragmatic breathing.

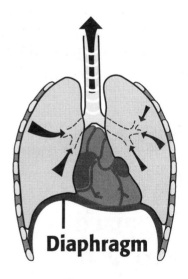

Diaphragm Relaxed:
air leaves the lungs,
organs move up and expand
as abdominal cavity relaxes

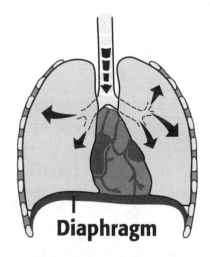

Diaphragm Contracted:
air enters the lungs,
organs compressed down
as abdominal cavity tightens

Abdominal breathing is awesome for a host of reasons: health, stress reduction, Chi or Ki cultivation, etc. But they do not relate to the narrow focus of *The Naked Warrior*: strength. Here is why diaphragmatic breathing is vital for strength.

Recall that inside your abdominal cavity are special sensors that measure the pressure inside your "spare tire." When the pressure goes up, so does your strength.

The downward pressure exerted by your diaphragm is essential for upping the IAP. Recall that when you "breathe into your stomach," the dome shaped muscle bears down and compresses your viscera. Breathing into your chest would pressurize your thoracic cavity and leave your abdomen weak; this does more to raise your blood pressure than your strength. So, breathe with your stomach, Comrade!

Inhale through your nose. Developing the habit so you keep your teeth in the ring is not the only reason. Taking your air in through a smaller hole will make for a stronger diaphragmatic action and better compression.

Note how sucking air in through your mouth creates a hollow, weak feeling inside. Now try it through your nose. To make an even stronger point, pinch your nose half shut and try it again. You cannot help noticing a powerful diaphragm action and a comfortable, strong feeling of compression.

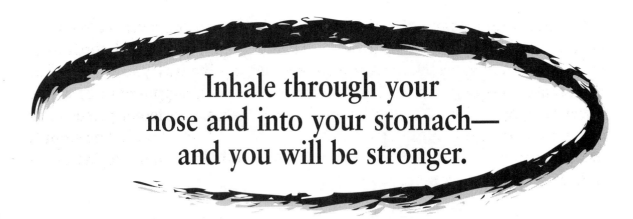

Inhale through your nose and into your stomach— and you will be stronger.

"Compression, not exhalation": a Tai Chi master demystifies Power Breathing

The most important thing you need to understand about power breathing is it is not really the breathing, the act of gas exchange between your lungs and the atmosphere that matters in strength amplification. It is the intra-abdominal pressure, or the compression. Breathing, in, out, or holding, is purely incidental to compression.

The martial arts world is not known for clarity of communication, which is why in many schools, students take years and decades to master the concepts they could have nailed in months or even weeks. A notable exception is tai chi master William C. C. Chen, who has some profound yet straightforward things to say about breathing:

"If you punch and exhale, you have no punch, you lose your energy…No professional fighters punch and exhale because they would lose their strength, have no compression and therefore no energy…Compression and making a sound is not exhaling; exhaling is different. Boxers punch and you hear them making the 'su' 'su' 'su' sound. That is not exhaling, that is compression. The difference between exhale and compression is that with compression you close the air valve; it becomes very small…When you exhale you are opening the valve and letting your air go out."

Do not misunderstand the above as an admonition to never let your air escape on effort! Some air will break through your closed vocal cords as if through a safety valve in a pressure cooker and it is the way you want it. But **the exhalation—or rather a very minor blast or air—is supposed to be a side effect of compression, not your intent!** Martial artists of different persuasions make all sorts of odd noises, "kiai," "wha," "hut," "sst," "pft". **The sounds are not the goal to strive for; making these sounds without trying is an indicator of proper compression.**

Think of your vocal cords as the nozzle on an air hose. When your vocal cords are relaxed, your air flows out freely, as it does with a passive exhalation, such as a sigh of relief. But when they close, it's a totally different ballgame. It's as if you have plugged the end of the hose with your thumb. Suddenly, very little air can escape—with noise—and the pressure inside the hose goes through the roof.

The former event, the glottis/nozzle open, the air flowing freely is what Chen calls exhalation. The latter, the glottis closed, is compression. Are you with me?

Bottom line, the breathing pattern is not as important as the compression or the IAP. In a Russian study the subjects' strength was compared during three different phases of breath: inhalation, breath holding, and exhalation. In a landmark slap to the Western gym beliefs, the exhalation group showed the lowest scores! The "inhalers" did better and the breath holders kicked everyone's butt.

The above does not mean that breath holding is the only way to go; there are multiple ways to achieve max compression once you understand power breathing. The point is, do not focus on where the air flows or does not flow; focus on the compression.

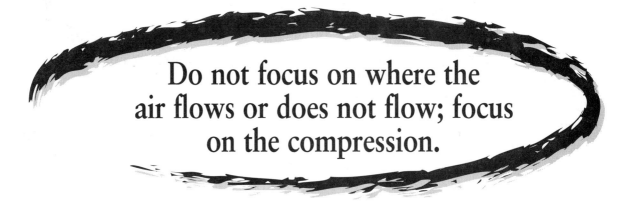

Do not focus on where the air flows or does not flow; focus on the compression.

Reverse power breathing: Evolution of the Iron Shirt technique

There are a number of ways to perform compressed breathing. A powerlifter friend of mine has a whole collection of noises that accompany his lifting: pneumatic or hissing, "mechanical" or buzzing, and "animal" or growling and grunting. He favors grunting for the deadlift, buzzing for the bench press, and hissing for curls.

While it may look complicated, it is not. **As long as the contents of your stomach are compressed—you are power breathing.** How you go about it is your business. And it does not even have to happen on an exhalation.

In my other strength books, I have explained the hissing version of power breathing and "virtual power breathing," or pretending to hiss but not letting the air come out. I will teach you a different compression technique in this book, reverse power breathing, which evolved from the traditional martial arts reverse breathing.

In my experience as an instructor, this is the quickest way to teach someone to pressurize. Why? Because it is similar to a body function you perform every day: a bowel movement. Forgive this distasteful analogy, but whenever you can recruit an old skill to a new skill, you will learn a lot faster.

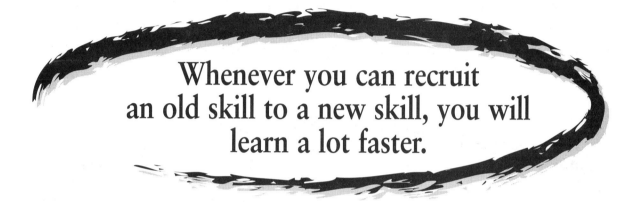

Whenever you can recruit an old skill to a new skill, you will learn a lot faster.

First, perform the anal lock. Contract your sphincter beforehand and keep your pelvic diaphragm pulled up whenever you have pressure in your abdomen from exertion. The anal lock is the standard operating procedure in many martial arts. This bizarre technique is vital for health and performance reasons.

Second, pretend that you are straining to have a bowel movement while maintaining the lock. Keep your face impassive. Don't try too hard the first time; just observe your body. You will notice a compression of your guts and a very powerful, stable feeling in your waist as your diaphragm anchors your torso. Your abdomen will slightly expand and so will your obliques.

It should be obvious that you should not practice reverse power breathing if you have a hernia.

Unless you are under a doctor's orders, don't fight the side expansion. It helps your strength, for a number of reasons. Don't let your stomach bulge, though; form a flat wall instead. Recall that the belly expansion happens as the result of your viscera being displaced by an aggressive diaphragm. The guts have to go somewhere, so they want to spread out and block the view of your shoes. Your abs should stop them.

Stand up. Brace your abs. Send the pressure low, very low, bear down. **"Not [to] the upper stomach,"** stresses Mas Oyama. **"Force it into the groin. Force the air down, down...Force your feet, if you are standing, or your seat, if you are sitting, right through the ground."**

Place your hands on your belly to make sure it stays flat. Brace your abs for a punch—flat and strong. Just don't mistake tightly flexed abs for a protruding stomach! If your six-pack is well developed, it will stick out somewhat. Your abs will bunch like a flexed bicep.

Lock your sphincter. The late Goju Ru karate master Yamaguchi supposedly got some heavy-duty hemorrhoids for failing to employ the anal lock during his dynamic tension Sanchin kata practice. The powerlifting community has its share of horror stories.

Lock and bear down. "Pack" your lower abdomen full of energy. As your diaphragm is pushing down trying to push out your viscera your abs and company should contain it with a "virtual belt." Do a couple of back-pressure crunches to refresh the skill of contracting your abdominals in a straight line.

To sum up: Pull up your pelvic diaphragm while bearing down or pushing down with your diaphragm. Contain the internal pressure with a tight midsection.

Go ahead and apply the reverse power breathing technique to the handshake. Your training partner won't like you!

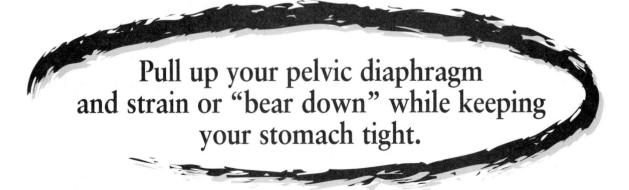

Pull up your pelvic diaphragm and strain or "bear down" while keeping your stomach tight.

Noticed how you have been breathing while practicing the compression technique? Probably not. Try again. What is it going to be? Have you been exhaling with a grunt? Or breathing shallow? Holding your breath? Or even inhaling on exertion? Which one is right?—All of the above. Remember the wisdom of William C. C. Chen: It is not the breathing but the compression that matters. Take care of the latter and the former will take care of itself.

But no matter how you breathe, remember two rules. First, if you choose to hold your breath, don't hold it longer than a couple of seconds. You can breathe shallow while staying tight for long exertions, such as isometric and dynamic isometric drills.

Second, don't take in too much or too little air. As Russian martial arts strength and conditioning expert V. N. Popenko has said, "A person must never have too much or too little air in his lungs." Having too much air prevents maximal tensing of the abdominal muscles, and having not enough air is just as bad. "When you exhaust your complete breath, a weak spot occurs," warned karate master Kanbun Uechi.

Oriental martial arts masters generally believe that you are at your strongest when you have expelled half of the air from your lungs. Russian research has found 75 percent to be ideal for strength. You don't need to worry about exact percentages. Just remember never to exhale or inhale all the way.

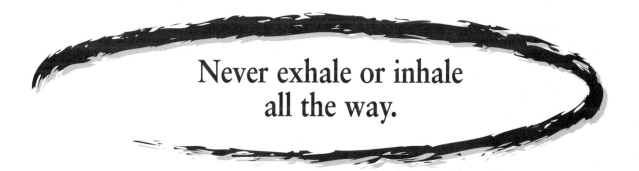

Never exhale or inhale all the way.

I'll wrap up this chapter with a post on the dragondoor.com forum. Here is what Marine, fighter, and powerlifting champ Dan "Garm" Bescher, RKC, says about reverse breathing:

"When one wants to express power, the most effective breathing pattern is an exhale where the abdomen moves outward—we see this in our lifting every day. In the context of internal martial arts, most reverse breathing is done in yang/hard gong. The grunt in the striking exercises quickly moves the abdomen out on exhale, and is designed to quickly move Qi from the Tantien to the area of the body upon which your mind is focused."

Power up from the core, or the "pneumatics of Chi"

Russian military hand-to-hand combat instructors emphasize two important principles of power generation: "summation" and "wave". Both refer to the skill of initiating an effort from the core of the body and then dynamically passing it along to the striking limb while adding force from every muscle along the way.

If any muscle along the power route fails to kick in, you have a "power leakage," in the words of Steve Baccari, RKC, a co-author of the *Power Behind the Punch* video. When that happens, your strength goes down the drain. That's as true for doing a one-arm pushup as it is in the boxing ring.

Whenever you exert yourself, always start tensing in your lower abdomen. Then send that tension outward to be amplified by the tension of the muscles closer and closer to the periphery.

Visualize how you are sending the pressure built up by the modified reverse breath along from your torso to your limbs, as if you are powered by pneumatics or hydraulics.

Imagine that your leg or arm is a long, thin balloon—the kind that clowns tie into knots to make animals. When you are at the bottom of the pistol or the one-arm pushup, the "balloon" is bent. "Blow it up" and it will straighten out.

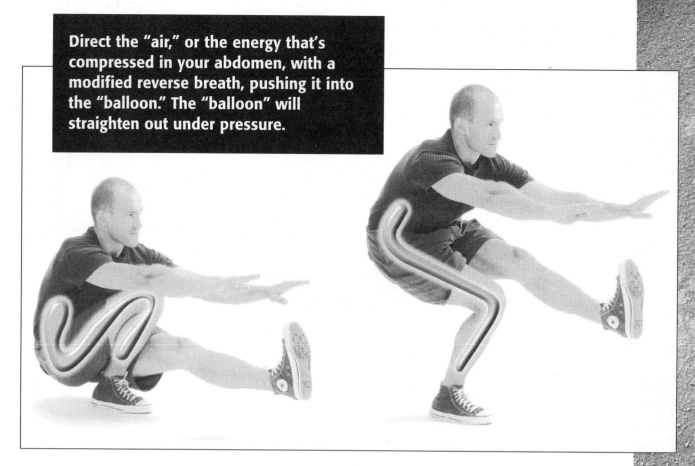

Direct the "air," or the energy that's compressed in your abdomen, with a modified reverse breath, pushing it into the "balloon." The "balloon" will straighten out under pressure.

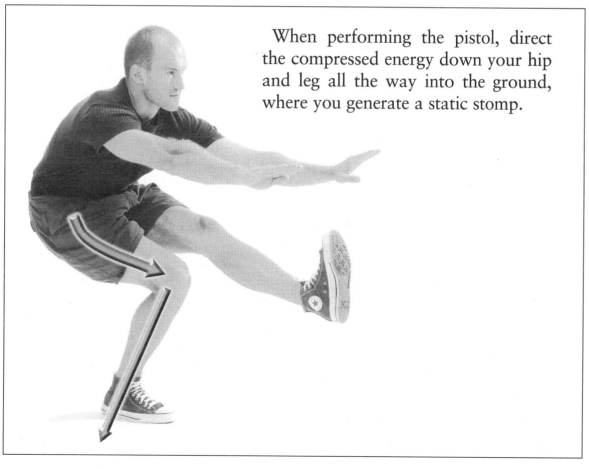

When performing the pistol, direct the compressed energy down your hip and leg all the way into the ground, where you generate a static stomp.

When performing the one-arm pushup, send the energy along your oblique and ribs, into your armpit, and then along your arm into your hand.

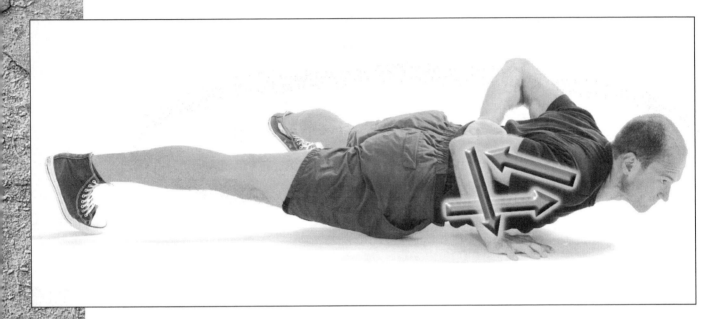

"The great power of the hips is concentrated and transmitted like chain lightning through the chest, shoulder, upper arm and forearm to the attacking surface of the fist," as Nakayama put it.

Make sure that the "balloon" reaches high enough to overlap your hip joint when doing the pistol and your shoulder joint when doing the one-arm pushup. You won't get very far with knee or elbow extension alone. Most power is generated closer to the core: the glutes in the pistol, the lats and pecs in the pushup.

Imagine that your arm or leg is a balloon that starts in your lower abdomen. When you are in the bottom position of the pistol or the one-arm pushup, the "balloon" has two kinks in it: at the hip and the knee and at the shoulder and the elbow, respectively. Direct the "air," or the energy that's compressed in your abdomen, with a modified reverse breath, pushing it into the "balloon." The "balloon" will straighten out under pressure.

I cannot overestimate the importance of proper breathing in power generation, be it in the gym or in the ring. You might find this a frustrating learning experience at times, but once you finally do get it you will have an awesome revelation of superpower.

"Fail to master breath control and you can do nothing in karate except possibly a few cute tricks," stated the late great Mas Oyama. Strength training is no different.

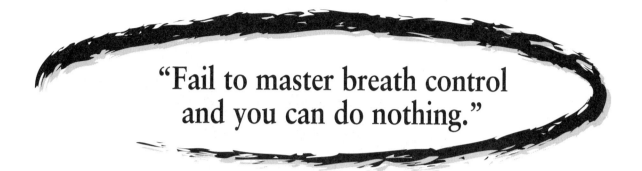

"Fail to master breath control and you can do nothing."

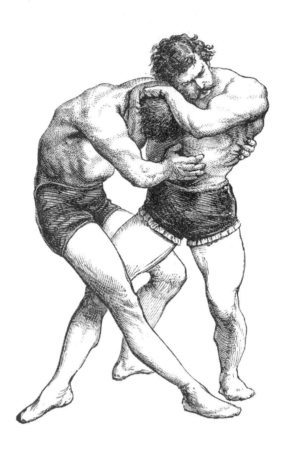

CHAPTER FIVE

DRIVING GTG HOME

• Driving GTG home: Focused
• Driving GTG home: Flawless
• Driving GTG home: Frequent
• Driving GTG home: Fresh
• Driving GTG home: Fluctuating
• Summing up GTG
• Summing up GTG even more
• Compressing GTG in ten words or less

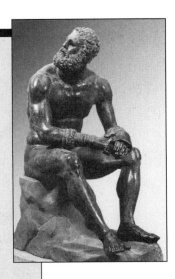

THE FIVE FS OF "GREASE THE GROOVE"

1. Focused
2. Flawless
3. Frequent
4. Fresh
5. Fluctuating

Driving GTG home: Focused

Kickboxing legend Bill Wallace took up fighting with one injured knee and he could kick with only one leg. So 'Superfoot' did twice as many kicks with his healthy one. He was one weapon short so he made his remaining weapon superior to his opponents' two. The rest is history.

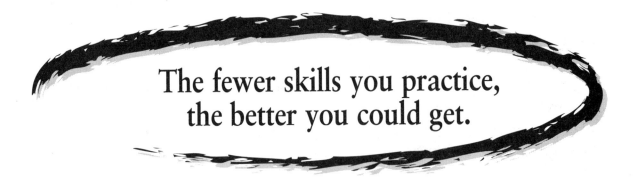

The fewer skills you practice,
the better you could get.

The "grooves" for different moves live and die by the laws of the jungle: they compete with each other. The fewer drills you practice, the better you are going to get.

Generally do not practice more than two unrelated exercises in the GTG manner. Follow a more conventional routine with less volume and frequency for other exercises should you decide to do them.

Driving GTG home: Flawless

Practice must be perfect. When it comes to max strength training, perfection, in addition to strictness of form, implies high muscle tension. Research by Russian experts such as Robert Roman clearly points to muscular tension, rather than fatigue, or reps, as the key to strength.

> Practice must be perfect.
> Max strength training perfection
> implies high tension.

High tension demands five conditions: significant external resistance, application of the High Tension and Power Breathing techniques, limiting the repetitions to five per set or less, approaching each set relatively fresh, and moving fairly slow.

Regarding "significant resistance," you do not have to live on a diet of max singles; this would burn you out in a hurry. But at least you should perceive the resistance as "moderately heavy".

The reps are slashed for the same cause of maxing the tension. Strength researchers have established beyond a shadow of a doubt that best "pure strength" gains are made when the repetitions are limited to five and under. Strength is a skill and skill practice must be specific. Low reps are specific to max strength. Do not rep out regular pushups if a one-arm pushup is your goal. Do not bother with Hindu squats if your goal is a one-legged squat or a pistol. I explain why in *Power to the People!* but no explanations should be necessary for this self-evident point.

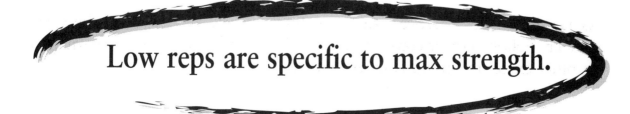

> Low reps are specific to max strength.

Driving GTG home: Frequent

"…there is no earthly reason why any man of a year's experience in weight training cannot perform [a bodyweight clean and military press]," stated Charles A. Smith in a 1947 issue of *Ironman*. I do not need to tell you that these days it is easier to find an honest biceps measurement than a bodyweight military press, even at a 'hardcore' gym.

Smith continues, "The reason why the records in the press have reached such astonishing heights…is because of this intensive application of specialized training in the press. [Russian champion] Novak presses every day, likewise [American champion] Davis…There is only ONE secret of success in pressing—and that is to press and press and press on each and every occasion you get near a bar. The record holders in the press actually use this method when they are in training to better their records."

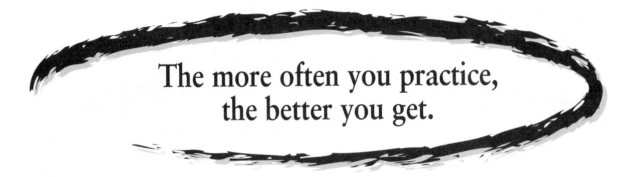

The more often you practice, the better you get.

It is elementary, Watson: the more you do something the better you get—as long as you avoid fatigue and overtraining. In a German study, training every other day delivered only 80% of the strength gains of daily training—and working out once a week yielded only 40%. It does not mean that you cannot train less frequently; you just will not gain as much strength.

Taking Sundays off is a good idea though. It will help you stay fresh. It is a good idea to stop your strength training a few hours before sleep as it has a tonic effect.

Driving GTG home: Fresh

Do as much as you can while staying fresh. It is a fine balancing act that requires discipline. Doing too little will slow down your progress. On the other hand, doing too much to the point where you get sore and weak, also sets you back. Listen to your body and err on the side of doing less rather than more.

Practice fresh and stop before your skill starts deteriorating. In other words, stop before you get tired.

"Remember, you should always feel stronger after your training than before you started. If you feel weak after a training session, you've overdone it." stated Midwestern strongman Steve Justa in *Rock, Iron, Steel: The Book of Strength*. If previous conditioning gives you trouble with this statement, just repeat: strength is a skill. Strength is a skill. Strength is a skill. And a skill is best practiced when you are fresh.

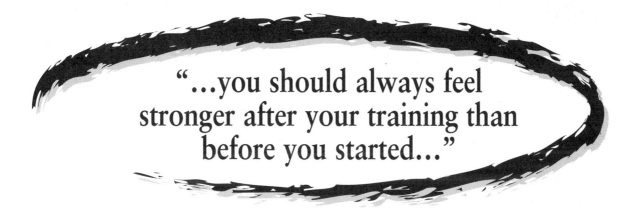

"...you should always feel stronger after your training than before you started..."

Freshness is another reason why low reps are preferred. Contrary to the bodybuilding mythology, low reps are easier to recover from. That means more frequent practice. That means more strength.

"Once I was in the performer's tent of a big circus, chatting with a very famous trapeze performer," recalled Charles MacMahon in his 1925 *The Royal Road to Health and Strength*. "Just before it was time for him to do his act, he walked over to a nearby ring, hooked the first and second fingers of his right hand around it, and chinned himself twice with his right arm. Then he did the same with his left arm. He did this to "warm up" for his performance, and he told me that it was all the exercise he took outside his performance; except when he had to practice for a new stunt. Everybody knows that it takes more strength to chin once with one arm that it does to chin twenty-five times with two arms. The funny thing is that it causes far less fatigue. The performer knew that, and that is why he was so economical of his time and energy."

Low reps are easier to recover from. That means more frequent practice. That means more strength.

Do not push to muscle failure or even close to it. Such balls to the wall training severely increases your recovery times and thus compromises your training frequency. There are other reasons to avoid failure. You learn what you practice. Why train yourself to fail? Practice to succeed! I have taken apart the flaws of training to failure in detail in *Power to the People!* should you care to know why.

Failure is not an option.

Most of the time do about half the reps you are capable of. Occasionally do less or more and come within a rep or two short of failure.

The balancing act between frequency and freshness is a tricky one. It requires listening to your body and patience in building up the volume and frequency. Instead of suddenly jumping into a routine of doing a set every hour every day, start with one or two easy sets a day. A few weeks later, add another set on alternate days. Then build up to three sets daily, etc. You get the idea: build up slow. Eventually your body will be able to handle an amazing workload—but it will not happen overnight.

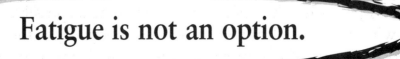

Fatigue is not an option.

Driving GTG home: Fluctuating

In order to get good at something you must practice it specifically.

On the other hand, if you keep doing the same thing you will eventually plateau.

So effective training must be different and the same simultaneously! A puzzle for a Zen master.

What is the answer to the koan?

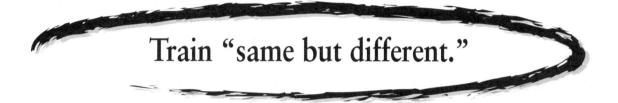

Train "same but different."

Practice variations of the same exercise. It is more effective, more fun, and less likely to develop overuse injuries.

Varying the sets, reps, proximity to failure, etc. also serves the purpose of keeping your training "same but different" for continuous progress. Russian lifters swear by this approach which they call 'waviness of load.'

It is better to do 10 total reps today, 30 tomorrow, and 20 the day after than 20 every day.

Marine vet Nick Nibler, RKC, has had great success with the "same but different" approach personally and with his "victims" at CrossFitNorth.com, a Seattle personal training gym he co-owns with Navy SEAL vet Dave Werner, RKC:

"I really wanted to hit the pull-ups hard…However, I didn't want an overuse injury or to have the training turn into mindless reps and sets that would quickly turn into a burden. So I decided to put a little variety in the program. I do pull-ups nearly every day now, but I try to never repeat the same workout twice. I put as much variety into the training as possible. I do weighted pull-ups with a kettlebell one day, use only bodyweight the next and sometimes perform many reps of assisted pull-ups with my feet in a loop of surgical tubing draped over the bar."

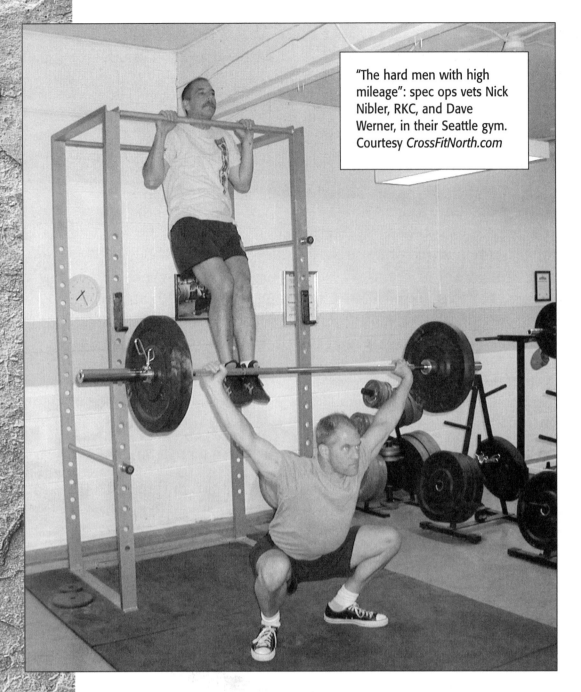

"The hard men with high mileage": spec ops vets Nick Nibler, RKC, and Dave Werner, in their Seattle gym. Courtesy *CrossFitNorth.com*

Note that the ex-jarhead mixes pure strength and strength endurance training. It works if you need both. If your focus is pure strength you should vary your reps in the one to five range. Remember, "different but the same."

"The intensity changes every day too. Sometimes I'll push it to my last good rep on every set and on other days I may only do 50-70% on each set for just a few sets. Ladders are great too. It is also useful to change the metabolic environment as well. Some days I'll try to stay as rested as possible between sets and space them out all day long. Mixed in to this there will be days when the pull-ups are part of a short circuit of exercises that I'll try to blow through as fast as possible. Another aspect that changes every day is the bar. I'll do pull-ups from a well supported bar, one that is wobbly, from a set of rings, from 2 hands on 1 rope and finally from 2 ropes hanging side by side. If the body needs a real change of pace, I get on the Concept 2 and row for a bit that day. This kind of active rest that works pulls in another plane has been very beneficial. I usually notice an increase in some aspect of my performance after a day or two on the rower. My work schedule and social obligations provide random days off so there is no need to plan those. They seem to come along at just the right time too.

"This approach to training has been very productive for me. My body never knows what is coming next and it seems to adapt very quickly to whatever training load it encounters. It is a very interesting program as well. Figuring out what variables I am going to focus on each day has turned the training into a game and kept it interesting. As for the pull-ups, I have never been able to do so many."

Listen to this hard man with high mileage.

Waving the load properly includes knowing when to cut back: if fatigue builds up or when you are about to test for a new PR.

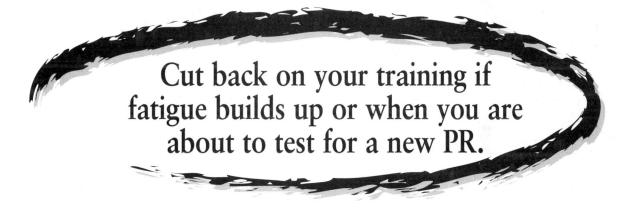

Cut back on your training if fatigue builds up or when you are about to test for a new PR.

Strength training and strength demonstration are not the same thing. The notion that you should break personal records every workout is nothing but a fairy tale. The less frequently you try for a PR, the better. Maxing every two weeks is a good guideline for beginners; every two months is more appropriate for experienced strength athletes. The elite should only try for PRs a couple of times a year.

And you should plan for it. A simple and effective taper is one or two easy days and one day off before a test. Using the 5RM pistol with a 53 lb. kettlebell as an example: your regular day, Tuesday might be 10x2@53lbs; Wednesday is the beginning of the taper with 5x2@36lbs; Thursday is an even easier day, 5x1@36lbs; with no negative, and Friday is a day off. On Saturday you should be able to put up six or even seven reps with a 53lb. kettlebell. You have gone over the five-rep limit and are ready for the 72-pounder!

Precede a strength test with one or two easy days and one day off.

Backing off is also in order if you have accidentally overtrained. If you are feeling tired, sore, and weak cut your volume or total weekly reps approximately in half until you are feeling fresh and raring to go. This is just a rough guideline; serious overtraining calls for more drastic measures.

Serious overtraining accompanied by symptoms such as overuse injuries or disturbed sleep is the result of stupidly refusing to listen to your body. Don't do it!

On the other hand, occasional mild overtraining is a lemon that can be turned into lemonade by an experienced strength athlete. "A river with a dam has more power," as a Lithuanian saying goes.

Back off immediately and you should see great gains, provided your overtraining is mild and you have backed off in time.

Some experienced strength athletes who are very attuned to their body purposefully push into slight overtraining and then taper and peak. Beginners are not advised to overtrain on purpose; it takes skill to pull out of a steep dive before crashing. But if you do accidentally do too much you will know what to do.

> "A river with a dam
> has more power."
> Mild overtraining followed by
> a taper might lead to great strength
> gains in experienced athletes.

Summing up GTG

- GTG pistols and one-arm pushups only. If you choose to do other exercises as well, train them separately on a more conventional routine
- Employ super strict technique
- Apply the High Tension and Power Breathing techniques
- Select exercise variations that feel "moderately heavy"
- Lift at a moderate to slow speed
- Limit the reps to five per set and less
- Strength practice six times a week, if possible in multiple mini-sessions, and take Sundays off
- Do not push to muscle failure or even close to it. Most of the times do about half the reps you are capable of. Occasionally do less or more and come within a rep or two of failure
- "…feel stronger after your training than before you started…"
- If you did overtrain slightly cut the volume by 50% volume until you are feeling fresh and raring to go
- Build up slow
- Practice variations of the same exercises. Constantly vary the sets, reps, and proximity to failure
- The less frequently you try for a PR, the better. Max every two weeks if you are beginners; every two months if you are an experienced strength athlete. Precede a strength test with one or two easy days and one day off

Summing up GTG even more

If you have the attention span of a ferret on a double espresso, here is the Reader's Digest version of "Grease the Groove."

- Only two exercises and their variations
- Moderately hard
- Tense
- Half the reps you are capable of, but no more than five
- At every chance, but never to fatigue

Compressing GTG in ten words or less

As the old Russian army joke goes, a sergeant is showing a squad of recruits around a tank. He says that there is a radio transceiver on the tank. A recruit asks, "Excuse me, sir, is the radio on transistors or microchips?"—"For the idiots I repeat: on the tank."

Here is the "tank version" of GTG. Brute strength does not get any more bare bone than this.

Minimize
- **The number of exercises**
- **Fatigue**

Maximize
- **Tension**
- **Frequency**

CHAPTER SIX

FIELD-STRIPPING THE PISTOL

- Box Pistol
- One-Legged Squat, Paul Anderson Style
- Airborne Lunge
- Pistol Classic
- Negative Free Pistol
- Renegade Pistol
- Fire in the Hole Pistol
- Cossack Pistol
- Dynamic Isometric Pistol
- Isometric Pistol
- Weighted Pistol

Marine Corps Martial Arts Program instructor trainer Sgt. Phillip Wyman knocks off rock bottom pistols with an 88-pound kettlebell. Clearly, you have some work to do. Here is your guide on taking your one-legged squat performance from zero to hero.

Box Pistol

The pistol comes in many flavors. The first variation to master is the box pistol, sitting back on a box or bench, rocking back, then rocking forward and standing up. The box squat has been hailed by many champion powerlifters, from George Frenn to Louie Simmons and Yuri Fomin, and for a good reason. For max squat power the quads are not enough; the glutes and the hamstrings must also be maximally recruited. The only way to make it happen is pre-stretching the hip muscles by sitting back rather than straight down. If this is done right, your shins will remain nearly vertical and your butt will protrude far back, almost as if you are doing a good morning.

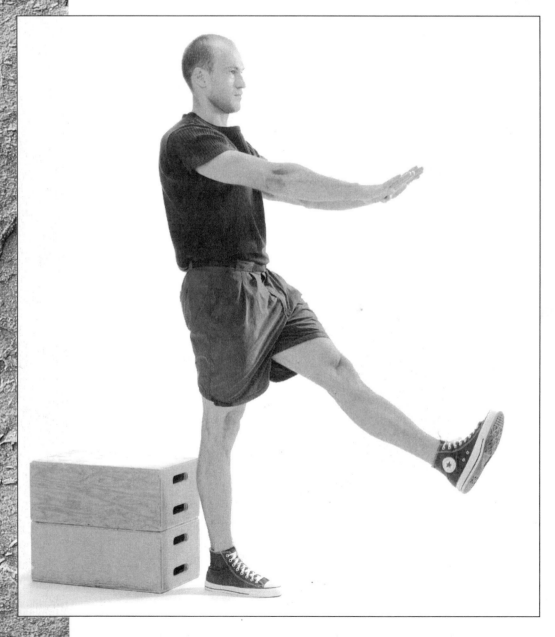

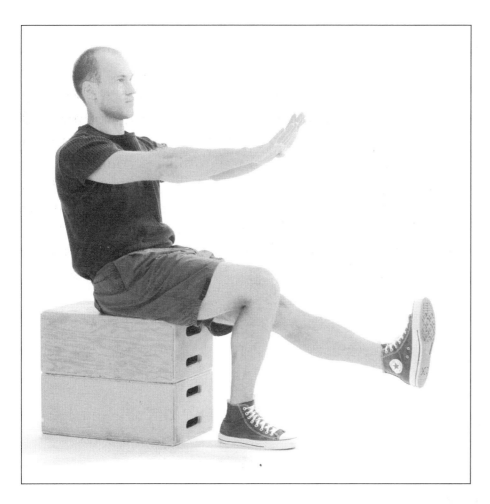

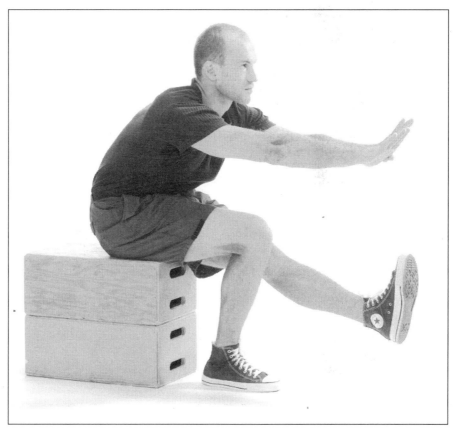

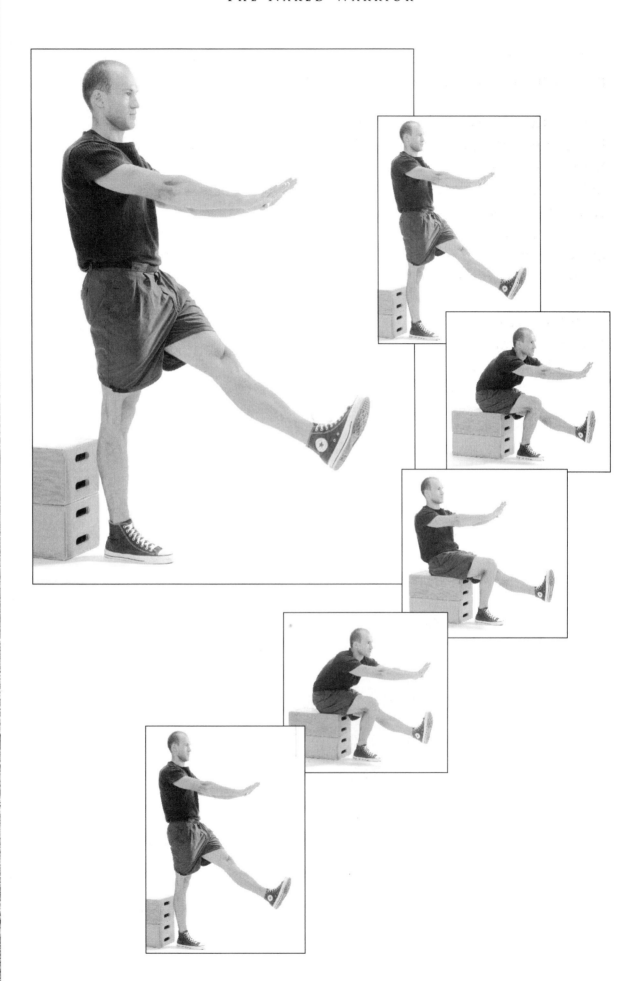

The reward will be remarkable squatting, jumping, kicking, and sprinting power, all around leg development, and low knee stress.

When the shin is kept nearly vertical the patella tendon is not smashing the kneecap into the joint. Besides, the knee is further protected from the rear by hamstring tension. It is a fact that the hammies stay tight all the way into the hole when you are box squatting by the book. That is rarely the case with conventional squats, at least for inexperienced squatters. No wonder powerlifters who had torn their patella tendons with traditional squats were known not to merely rehab themselves with box squats but to make a quantum leap in their total—without any further knee problems!

Another reason the box variation of the one-legged squat is so great is the ease of adaptation to any strength level. While the rocking squat off the floor is even harder than the regular rock bottom pistol, a pistol to a high bench is within anyone's ability. As you get stronger just increase the depth.

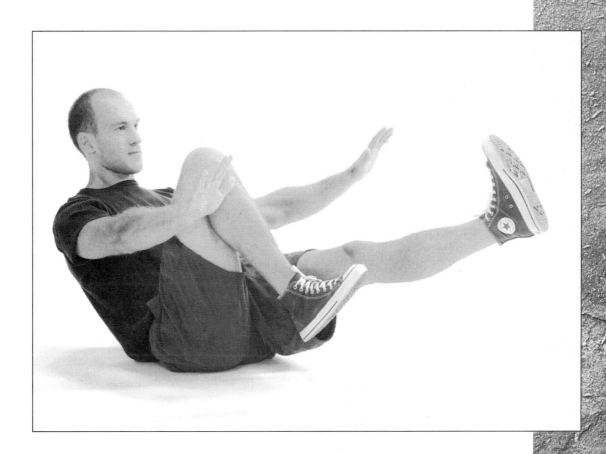

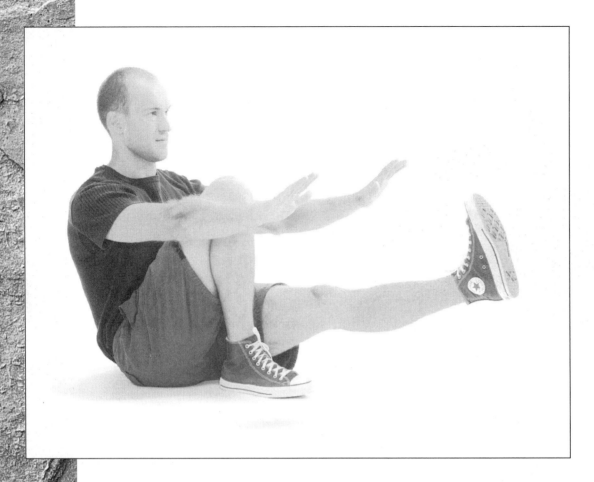

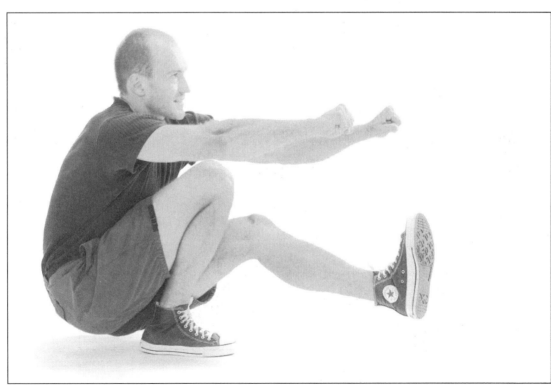

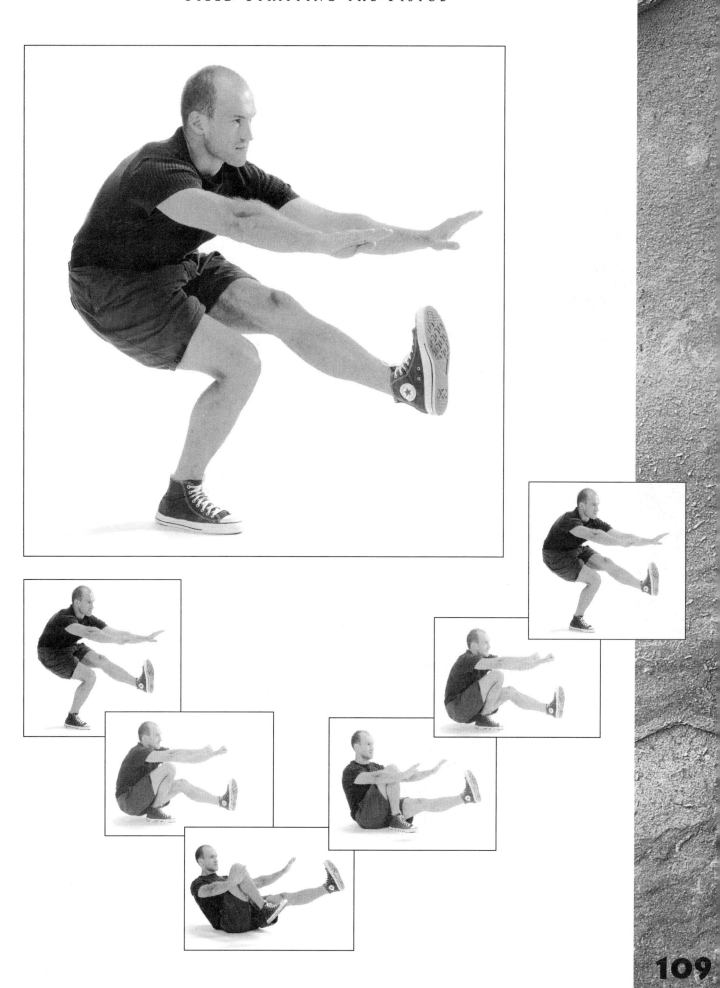

Touch and go without rocking is another way to do it. Completely relaxing before flexing off is the most evil option.

Stand a couple of feet in front of a box set high enough to stop you at a quarter squat. Go barefoot or wear flat shoes: Chuck Taylors, wrestling shoes, etc. Pistols are easiest in boots, so boots may be a good starting point. Fancy cushioned sneakers are no good. Use the simple rule of thumb: the more you paid for your shoes, the less suitable they are for strength training.

Lift one nearly straight leg in front of you, and squat. Make a point of keeping your weight on your heel and sticking your butt out as far as possible—think a good morning, not a squat. Keep your arms in front of you for balance. You may find that holding a light weight, say a five or ten pound plate, will help with balance. With or without weight, reach forward as far as possible—without letting your knee slip.

As Rob Lawrence, RKC Sr., put it, "You have to lean forward as much as you do in a good morning. If you don't you will lose your balance and fall backwards. Think about it: when you are standing straight up you are perfectly balanced. If part of you goes backward, an equal part of you must go forward or you will fall over."

"To make sure you are leaning forward enough, I recommend keeping your head in line with your support foot as you descend. In fact, when you start out you can even look right down at the foot. Since you are not carrying weight on your back as in the squat, this is not dangerous."

"Pretty soon you will notice, if you lean forward enough in order to counterbalance your sitting back, you will descend successfully. If you don't lean forward enough, you will fall backwards."

Mas Oyama used to make an amusing demonstration of physics relevant to the box pistol. He would have a student sit in a chair and press just one finger against the student's forehead. The karate master would instruct the latter to get up and the student could not as his center of gravity was behind his feet. Take notice.

It is imperative that your knee does not buckle in and does not hang over your toes; the closer to vertical is your shin, the better. Pretend that you are stuck in cement up to your knee or are wearing stiff ski boots. Do wear ski boots if you must.

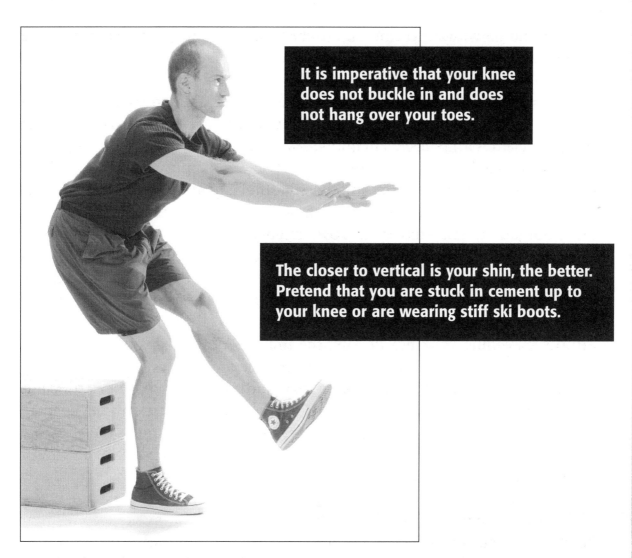

It is imperative that your knee does not buckle in and does not hang over your toes.

The closer to vertical is your shin, the better. Pretend that you are stuck in cement up to your knee or are wearing stiff ski boots.

Sit back with control, rock back until you are upright. Rock forward—far forward—without hesitation and stand up, explosively, but without losing tension.

You will notice that you have a tendency to shift your foot underneath you the moment before you stand up. Your quad is so dominant that you subconsciously want to shift all the work to it and unload your weak ham and glute. Don't! Go on a higher box if necessary but achieve a vertical shin and a foot that is "glued" to the floor!

One technique that will help you keep your lower leg upright is to have your training partner place his or her hand on your shin an inch or two below your kneecap. The partner will physically stop your shin from moving forward should you go against the Party directive.

Be sure to contract your glute when you are standing up. "Pinch a coin" with your cheeks. Once more: stay on your heel.

Once you have gotten the hip thrust action down pat and you are comfortable squatting to a high box you will have other things to worry about. As the depth of your rocking pistol increases, you will notice that it is virtually impossible to go deeper than a couple of inches above parallel without letting your knee slip forward. I am sure you have experienced the same problem with barbell squats.

No big deal, just use a tip from powerlifters: instead of yielding to the weight, actively pull yourself into the hole with your hip flexors, the muscles on top of your thigh. Here is how to recruit them. Lie on your back and pull your leg towards your chest, as high as you can, against mild resistance from your training partner. Try to get the same feeling when you are descending into a squat; literally pull yourself down with the hip flexor.

In the beginning your hip flexors, the muscles on the tops of your thighs, might cramp a bit, especially on the airborne leg. Stretch them between sets by lunging or kneeling on one knee and pushing your hips forward while keeping your torso upright. Do very few sets and reps until you adapt—which might take weeks.

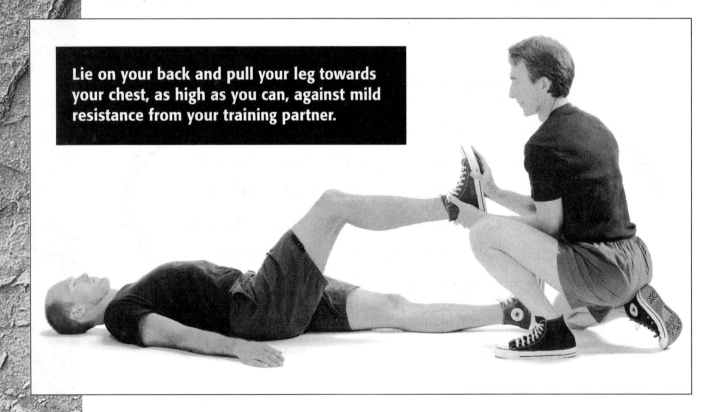

Lie on your back and pull your leg towards your chest, as high as you can, against mild resistance from your training partner.

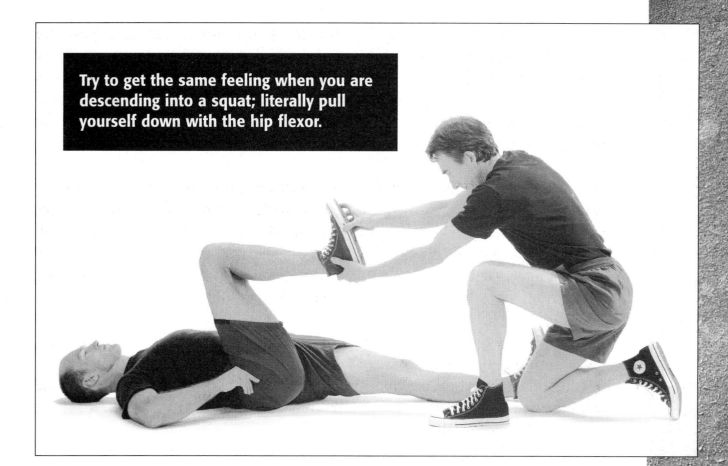

Try to get the same feeling when you are descending into a squat; literally pull yourself down with the hip flexor.

The hip flexor muscles on top of your thigh below the abdomen are easy to overwork with pistols! Make sure to stretch them after every set and to build up your volume very gradually!

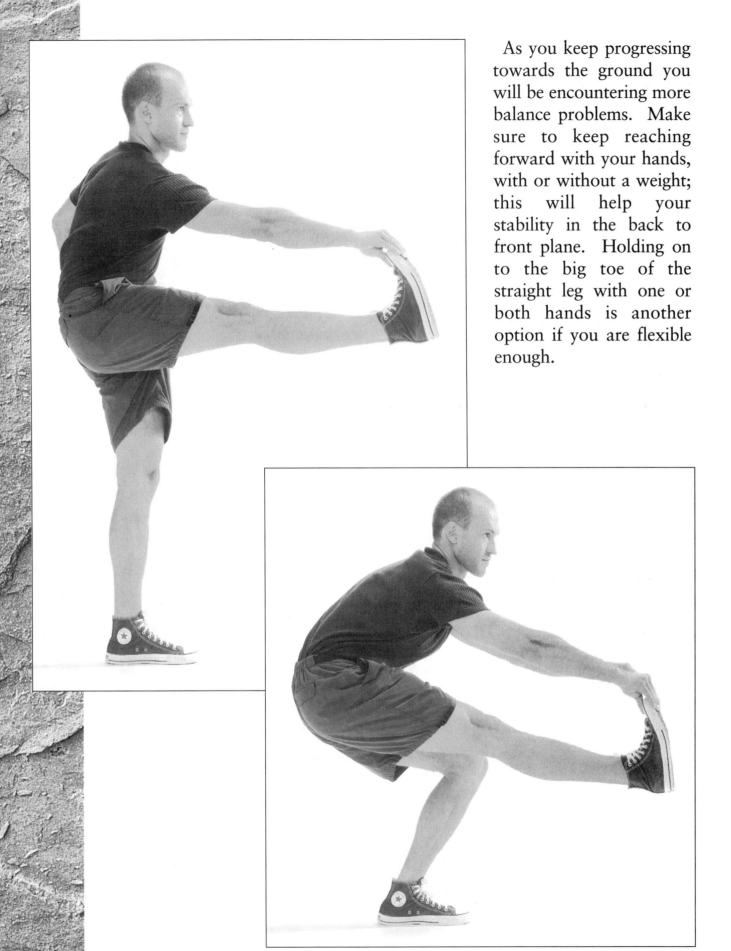

As you keep progressing towards the ground you will be encountering more balance problems. Make sure to keep reaching forward with your hands, with or without a weight; this will help your stability in the back to front plane. Holding on to the big toe of the straight leg with one or both hands is another option if you are flexible enough.

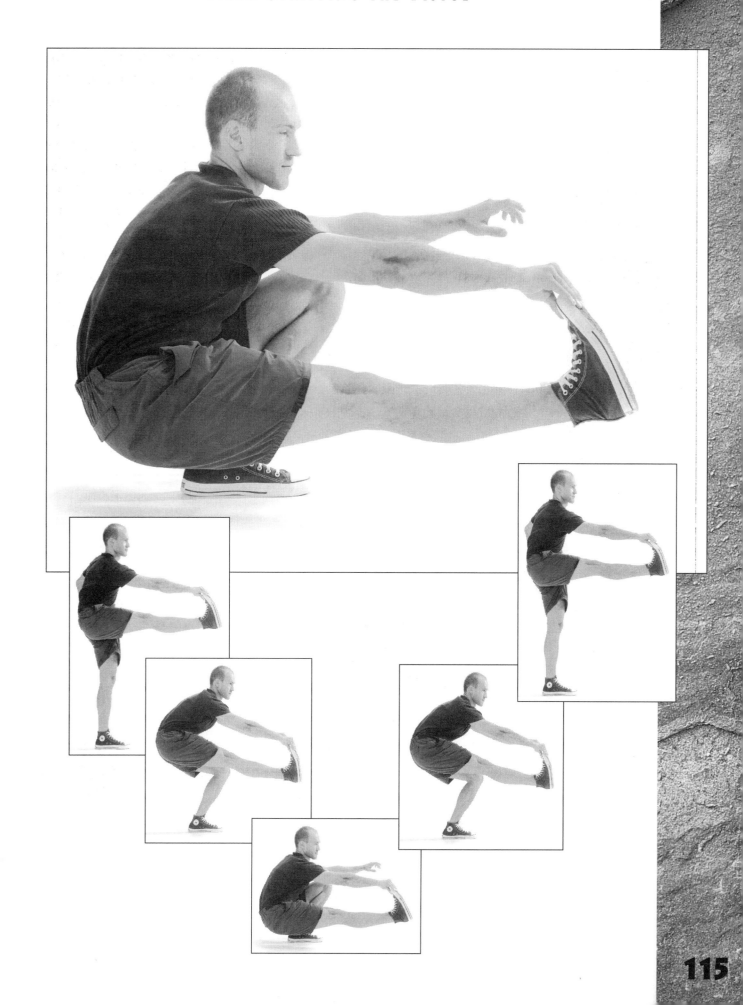

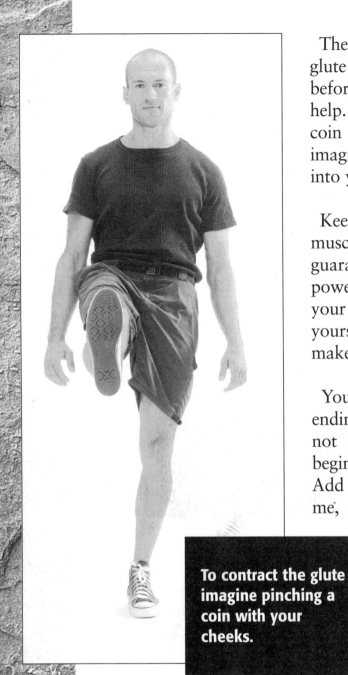

To contract the glute imagine pinching a coin with your cheeks.

The side-to-side balance is tougher. Flexing the glute and the inner thigh of the squatting leg before you start descending is going to be a big help. To contract the glute imagine pinching a coin with your cheeks. To flex the adductors imagine "zipping them up" from your knees up into your groin.

Keep these muscles—and the rest of the leg muscles!—tight as you go down and you are guaranteed to have better balance and greater power. Another cool tip is to grip the deck with your toes. And yes, it is okay to slightly help yourself with your other leg in the beginning. Just make sure to wean yourself off ASAP.

You may be getting exhausted from the never-ending details by now. Be patient. First, you do not have to apply them all at once, in the beginning just keeping your shin vertical will do. Add new power tips as the weeks go by. Trust me, it is worth it. Gains do not come from complex routines; they come from simple ones that pay attention to details. "It took me FOREVER to do pistols correctly," admitted Rob Lawrence, RKC Sr., on the dragondoor.com forum. "It was worth every ounce of effort."

Gains do not come from complex routines; they come from simple ones that pay attention to details.

More details. Inhale on the way down or when you are on the box. The moment your butt is about to clear the box pressurize your abdomen. Your waist will feel powerfully tight. The 'Chi' generated will flow into your working leg and you will stand up with no effort! Personally, I prefer the hissing version of power breathing for pistols, but it is just one legit option.

Once you have worked down to a very low, curb level, rocking pistol keep moving down until you sit back on the deck! Visualize punching straight through the ground with your heel when you are standing up. The action is similar to the taekwondo back kick. The foot of your working leg will lift off the ground as you are rocking back. This unloading—you may try it at higher levels too—will make the squat very tough. So tough that the regular rock bottom pistol will feel like a piece of cake!

Some comrades' builds will not allow them to do a deck pistols; if you cannot keep your balance even with good flexibility you will have to hold a weight in front of you.

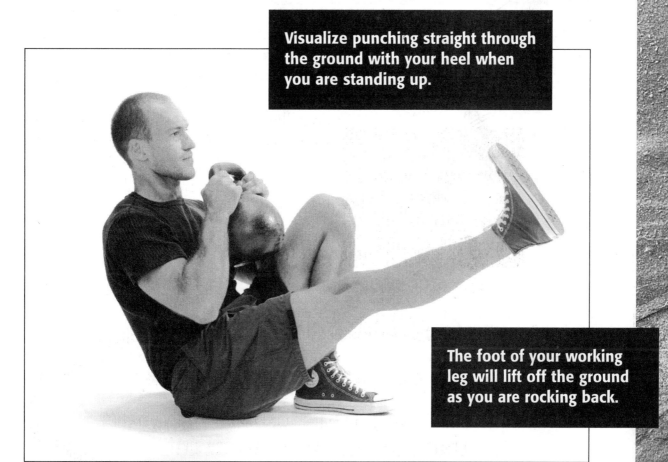

Visualize punching straight through the ground with your heel when you are standing up.

The foot of your working leg will lift off the ground as you are rocking back.

A Progressive Box Pistol Workout Inspired by Paul Anderson

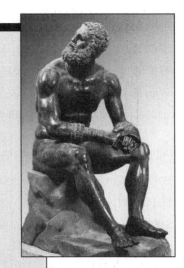

Do a set of rocking pistols to a high box a rep or two short of failure. One leg, then, after a minute or so, the other. Your reps will be higher than five; it is all right as the distance is shorter than usual.

Lower the box level by an inch or two and do another set. Stretch your hip flexors lightly between your sets to prevent them from tightening up. Keep progressing in this fashion until you are down to one rep, then work back up. You will be a hurting unit!

One-Legged Squat, Paul Anderson Style

Paul Anderson did include one-legged squats in his power regimen. He did not do pistols with his free leg in the front though, probably because of his girth. So "the Wonder of Nature," as Russians called him, would stand on a table with his free leg hanging and hold on to something for balance. The free leg remained straight throughout; the table had to be tall enough. "A picnic table works great for this exercise," explains Brazilian Jiu Jitsu World Champion Steve Maxwell, RKC Sr., on the dragondoor.com forum.

"I have also used various other pieces of furniture such as desks, heavy tables, tree stumps and even a dresser once. I think this movement is a great alternative to pistols. The working hip and thigh gets a complete range of motion. Flexibility is not an issue as in the pistol and a lot of weight crushing down on the neck and shoulders is not necessary to work the hip and thigh muscles. Even though I can do pistols with no problems, I still use this exercise as an alternate especially when wearing a weight vest. The weight vest tends to pull me off balance backwards when performing my pistols. When I am moving from pullups, dips, or pushups to my one leg squats with compressed rest periods, it is a hassle taking the vest on and off to do the pistols. I just jump up on my dining room table with my vest on and crank out one legged squats (only when my wife is not home). It's easier to keep my balance with the vest on when I can dangle my leg. I don't like holding on to something for balance because I find it to easy to cheat."

This one-legged squat variation, if practical, is an excellent addition to your regimen. You can handle a higher volume of squats because your hip flexors do not have to hold your leg up.

Airborne Lunge

Here is another easier variation of the one-legged squat. Keep your free leg in the air behind you, semi-bent. Squat down until your knee—but not your foot!—touches the deck and get back up. It helps to reach forward and fold over as if you are doing a good morning. Make sure that your heel stays planted. It goes without saying: do not bang your knee into the floor.

This drill is easier than the pistol but it is not as easy as it looks. Make sure that your rear foot completely clears the deck to appreciate it.

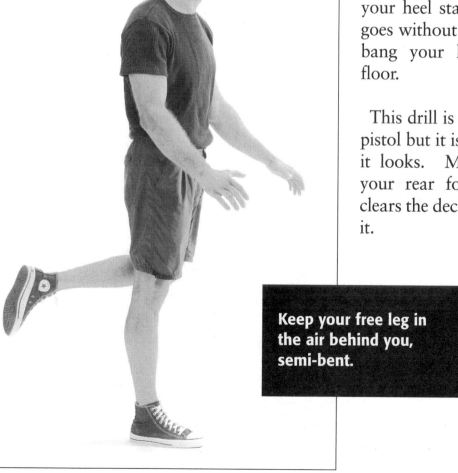

Keep your free leg in the air behind you, semi-bent.

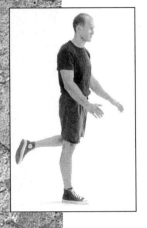

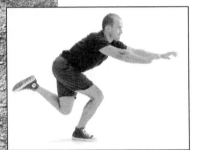

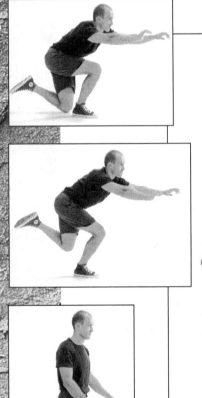

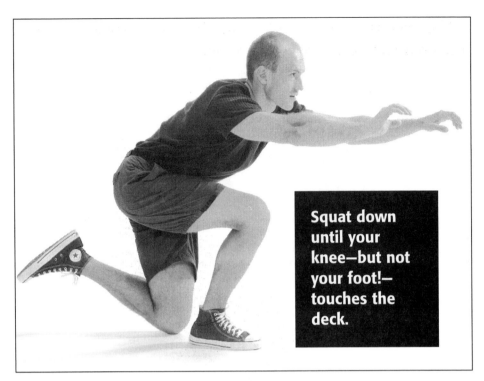

Squat down until your knee—but not your foot!—touches the deck.

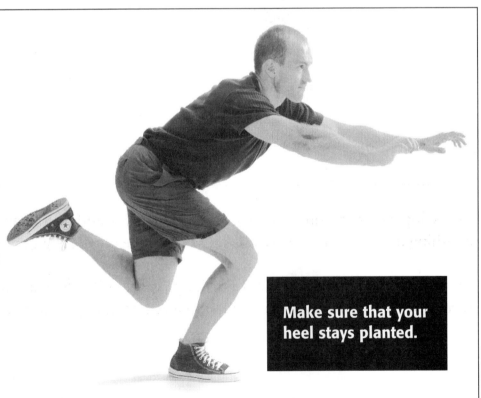

Make sure that your heel stays planted.

The exercise can be made easier by sliding something under your knee and thus reducing the range of motion.

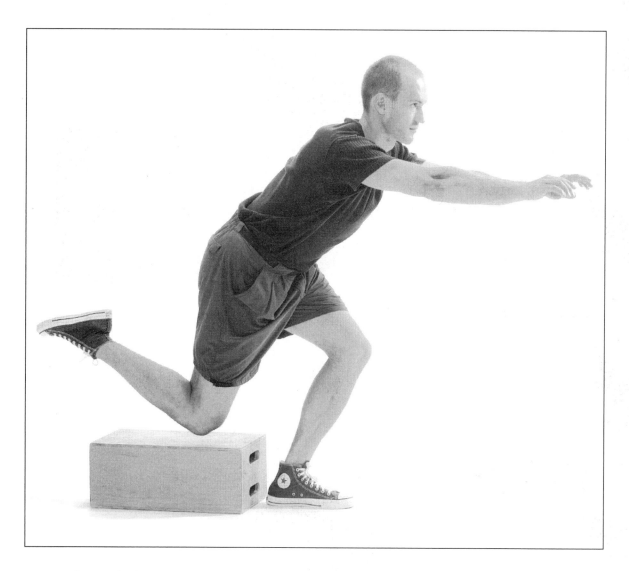

It is logical that you can make it harder by standing on an elevation but anything above an inch or two is not a good idea; too rough on your knee.

If you want to make the airborne lunge more difficult pause and relax for a second with your knee on the ground before tightening up and heading back up.

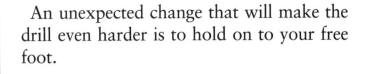

An unexpected change that will make the drill even harder is to hold on to your free foot.

This drill is easier than the pistol but it is not as easy as it looks. Make sure that your rear foot completely clears the deck to appreciate it.

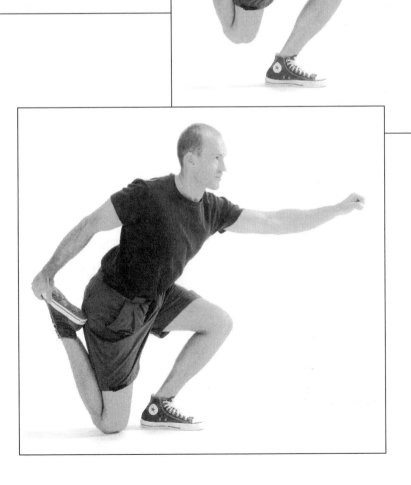

Pistol Classic

At last, the real deal.

Go rock bottom and get up without bounce. Easier said than done. Before attempting the classic pistol you need enough balance and flexibility to comfortably stay in the rock bottom position. In the beginning you may hold a very light, five to ten pound weight far in front of you for counterbalance. Do not hold on to anything else; it is too easy to cheat!

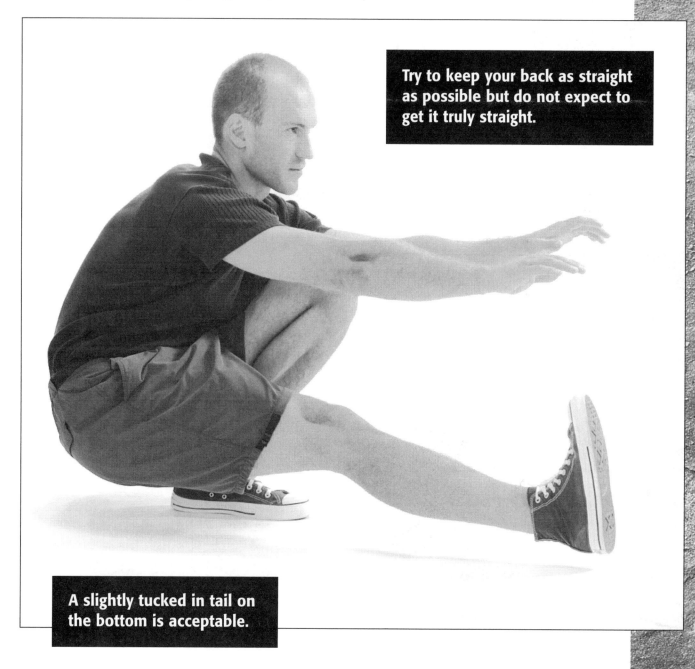

Try to keep your back as straight as possible but do not expect to get it truly straight.

A slightly tucked in tail on the bottom is acceptable.

To do the conventional one-legged squat pull yourself in the hole as you have for the rocking squat but instead of sitting on the deck sit on your haunches. Try to keep your back as straight as possible but do not expect to get it truly straight. Unless you have medical restrictions, a slightly tucked in tail on the bottom is acceptable.

Understand the difference between "straight" and "upright". "Upright" is a physical impossibility with the heel planted unless you have the ankle flexibility of a mutant. Go for "straight", in other words "not rounded."

Pause long enough to eliminate the bounce. This makes the drill both harder and safer. Pressurize your abdomen and pop up. Stand up all the way, make sure to stretch your hip flexors by aggressively driving your hips forward.

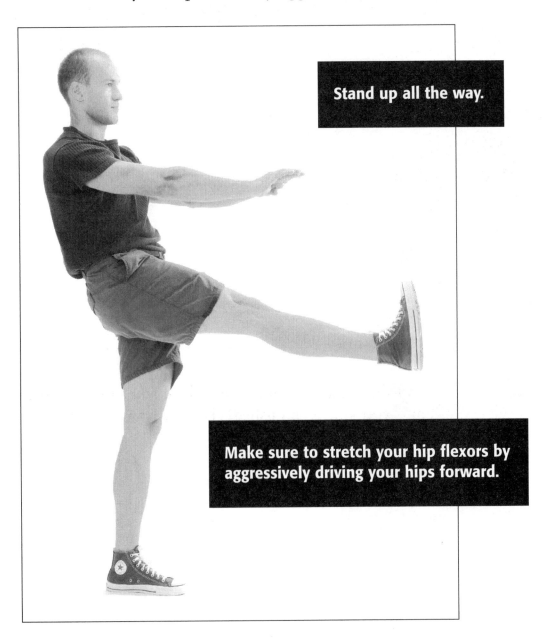

Stand up all the way.

Make sure to stretch your hip flexors by aggressively driving your hips forward.

As before, do not let your knee slip forward or bow! An effective technique for learning to keep your shin nearly vertical and to drive from your heel is to do your one legged squats off a barbell plate or a similar elevation. NOT by elevating the heel the way bodybuilders do it, but by placing the back half of your foot on the plate and letting your toes hang in the air.

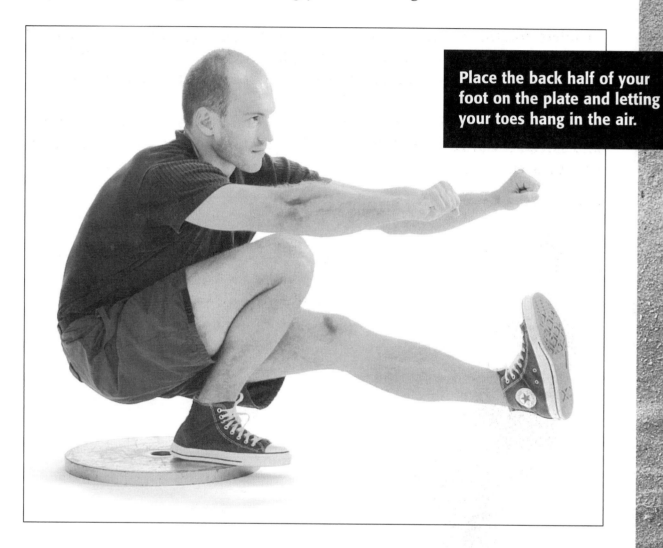

Place the back half of your foot on the plate and letting your toes hang in the air.

As soon as you cheat and shift your weight to the balls of your feet your toes will touch the ground and you will be punished! Do not let your knee bow in, your ankle cave in, or your body rotate.

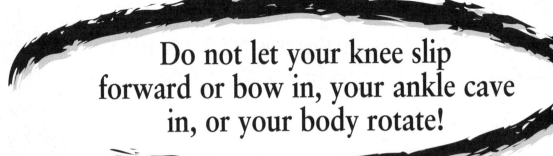

Do not let your knee slip
forward or bow in, your ankle cave
in, or your body rotate!

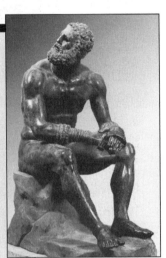

AN OLYMPIC WEIGHTLIFTER'S GETTING-STARTED TRICK

Sixty-two year old hard man J. D. Wilson posted this on the dragondoor.com forum, "Get comfortable in the bottom position [of the pistol]. I stole this idea from Gary Valentine who has published some great ideas on learning Olympic lifting on the Old School Strength Training site...practice a static hold in the bottom position...The object? If you can't handle this position with ease and comfort (using a light weight), how do you think you'll do when you catch something real (i.e. heavy) in the same position?

"So, I've been doing the same thing in the bottom position of the pistol. In truth, I lack the flexibility to hold a static pose at the bottom and need to hold some weight in front...to maintain the position. It's a combination stretch and balancing act. Relax into it!"

When relaxing into the stretch let out sighs of relief; imagine that you are letting the air and energy/tension out through your hip and knee.

DO YOU HAVE A HARD TIME KEEPING YOUR FREE LEG UP AND STRAIGHT? —HERE IS ANOTHER SOLUTION FROM THE PARTY

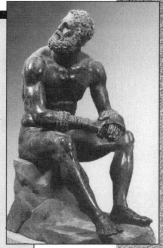

"My quads on the lifted leg have to strain very hard to keep the leg even close to straight. Obviously, stretching is the solution (though I like tight hams for lifting). Anyone who wanted to excel in pistols might benefit from some extra hamstring flexibility," stated Dan Bescher, RKC.

Even if you have sunk into a full squat you may still have a flexibility problem with keeping your free leg airborne. "Do what the yogis do when they aren't flexible or strong enough to perform a pose correctly—use a prop," suggested James 'Lemon' Boelter on the dragondoor.com forum. "Get yourself a Theraband/Jump Stretch type of tube or a length of rope of the correct length; wrap one end around your instep, the other to your waist/hips/neck (whatever seems to work without cutting off your circulation); the rope should be tight enough to lend some upward 'pull' to help your leg extend."

LEARNING HIP DRIVE FROM A FULL CONTACT FIGHTING CHAMPION

If you have read my abs book or have used the Ab Pavelizer™ you can take advantage of the awesome tip by pistol mutant Steve Cotter, RKC Sr. This full contact champ suggested that you imagine that you are performing a Janda situp on one leg. Do not forget to grip the deck with your toes at the same time. The motion is somewhat similar to 'pawing' the ground while pushing off the starting block for a sprint. The power and tension is awesome!

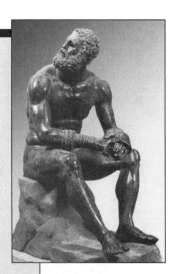

CANADIAN KETTLEBELL INSTRUCTOR'S VISUALIZATION FOR STRONGER AND BETTER BALANCED PISTOLS

Even when you are not holding a weight it may be a good idea to imagine that you do. "Pretend you are holding a kettlebell in your hands," suggested Pietro Puzzuoli, RKC, on the dragondoor.com forum. "This will ensure you keep your abs and whole upper body tight, which will add tension to your quads. Also, holding an imaginary KB forces you to learn proper balance w/o the need of artificial aids like chairs or doorways."

Keep in mind that as any power tool, the pistol can be dangerous. Follow all the fine points to the 'T' and do not try a variation you are not ready for!

As with any power tool, the pistol can be dangerous. Follow the instructions and use your head!

Negative-Free Pistol

Comrade, have you tried concentric-only training? That is, strength exercises that de-emphasize the negative. There are at least three reasons to do it. One, to build strength without building muscle mass. Two, to up the loading volume without overtraining. And three, to increase or maintain strength while avoiding muscle soreness and maximizing recovery. 1,000 pound squatter Dr. Fred Hatfield recommends this technique to powerlifters peaking for a meet.

Squat rock bottom on both feet and slowly bring one leg forward. Compress your abdomen, tense your whole body, and get up on one leg. It works just as well for box pistols.

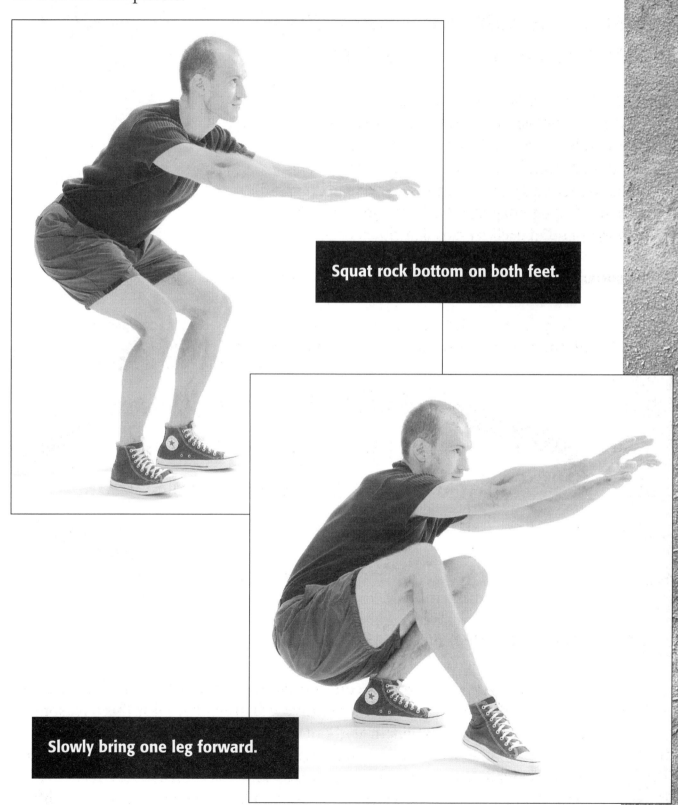

Squat rock bottom on both feet.

Slowly bring one leg forward.

129

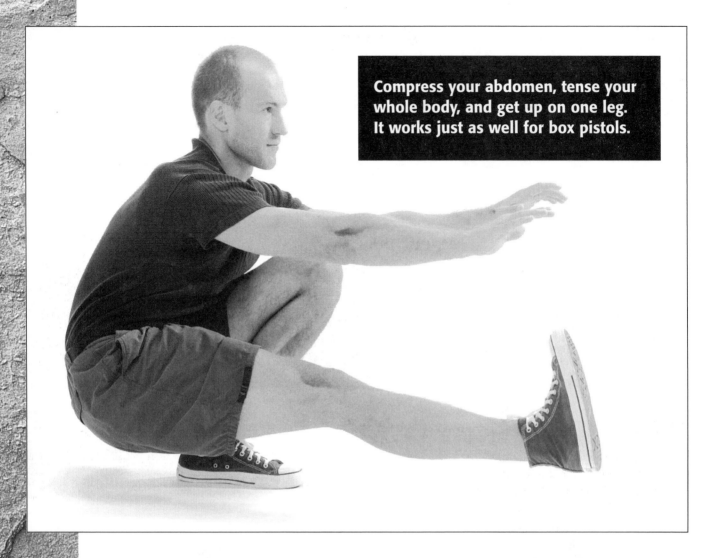

Compress your abdomen, tense your whole body, and get up on one leg. It works just as well for box pistols.

Some comrades with tweaked knees will like the low knee stress of negative free pistols. Whenever my torn MCL acts up I just practice concentric only one-legged squats with no pain whatsoever.

You may even start your pistol training with this variation. Many people have a hard time getting down safely in the beginning, unable to fire their hip flexors and apprehensive about losing balance and falling. A little hairy for the knee. But once you have successfully stood up you should have no problem coming back down in the groove you have made on the way up.

All-Around Lifting National Champion and Record Holder Andy Komorny, RKC, made a suggestion brilliant in its simplicity, on working the concentric-only box pistol into your day on the dragondoor.com forum: "Every time you get up from your chair, do it on one leg...shin vertical and weight on the heel."

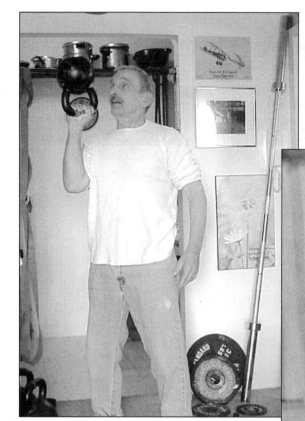

Andy Komorny, RKC, on his seventieth birthday. *Photo courtesy Andy Komorny*

Andy Komorny doing a different kind of squat. "Here's me doing a 100 kilo [222 pounds] Steinborn lift for a record at the 2002 All-Around Weightlifting World Championships. The photographer didn't get the squat portion. You get the bar up on your back from the floor, squat, and then put it back to the floor."
Photo courtesy Andy Komorny

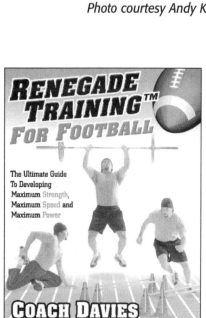

Renegade Pistol

Coach John Davies, RKC, the author of *Renegade Training for Football*, suggested the following advanced pistol variation on the dragondoor.com forum. Lower yourself on one leg. Then slowly switch feet without help from your hands and without sitting down. Stand up on the other leg and then reverse the drill.

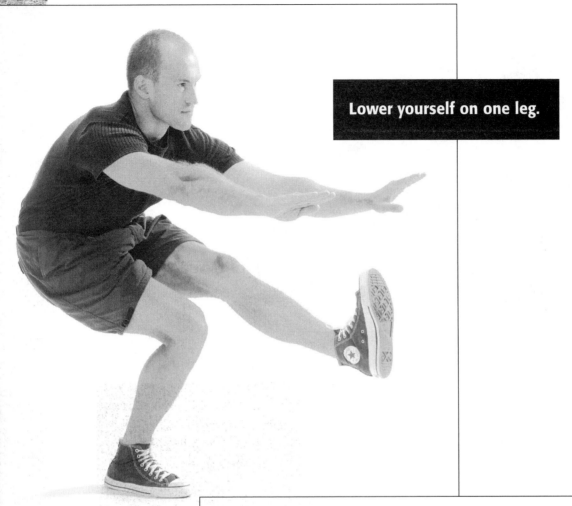

Lower yourself on one leg.

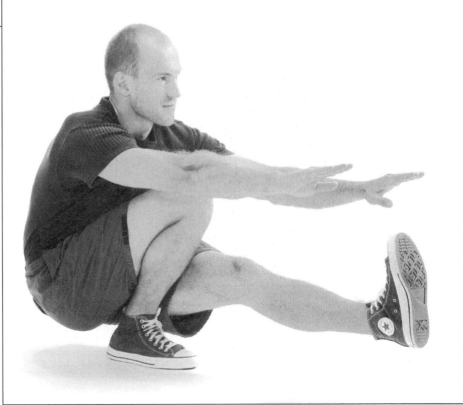

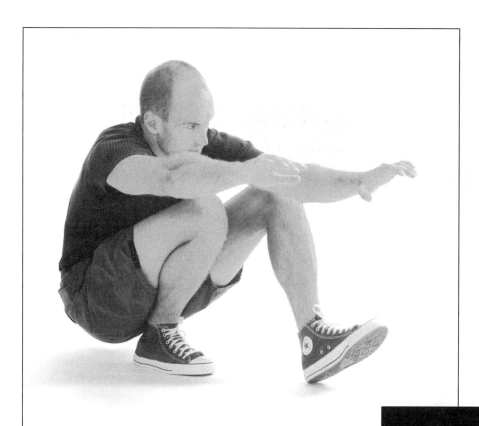

Then slowly switch feet without help from your hands and without sitting down.

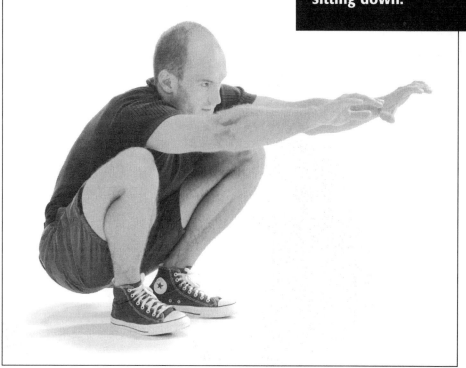

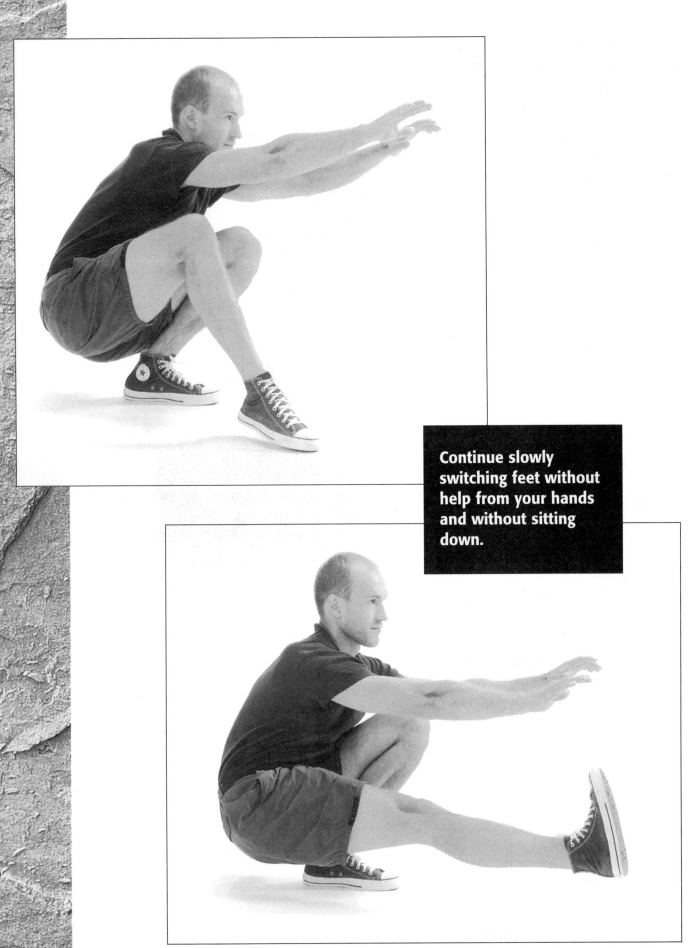

Continue slowly
switching feet without
help from your hands
and without sitting
down.

The exercise can be done explosively; just remember not to compromise tension for speed! Accelerate out of the bottom and jump. Land on the other foot, descend slowly, switch feet on the bottom slowly, and jump again.

Until you rule the pistol classic—forget about it!

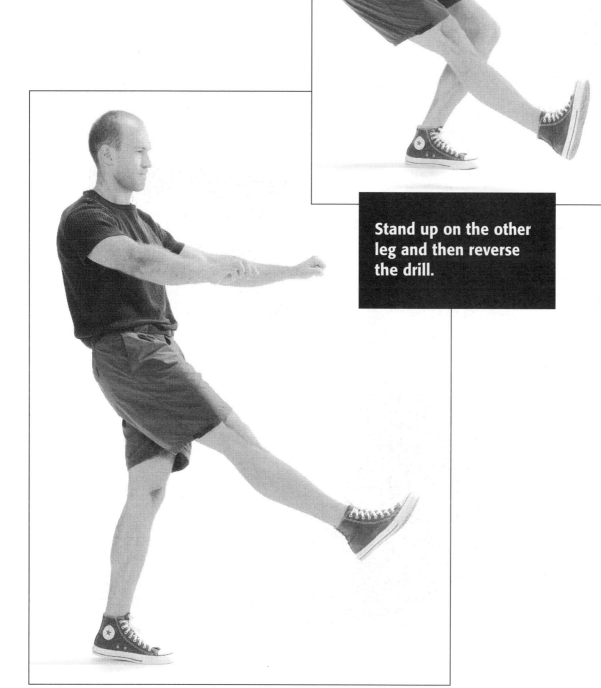

Stand up on the other leg and then reverse the drill.

135

Fire-in-the-Hole Pistol

"I was working on pistols the other day," posted Tom Furman, RKC, on the dragondoor.com forum. "I sat on the ground, pulled my knee up to my chest/shin vertical, and extended leg locked. I held a kettlebell with my hands"—a weight is optional—"and tried to brace and FIRE my hamstring, adductors, glutes, hip flexors with lots of abdominal tension. I did not pop up and bounce hamstring against calf affecting my knee integrity, but powered up and down a few inches with some control. This is a good drill to do with a weight that you cannot lift in the pistol exercise. Low reps like 3 per side, switching and resting seems to be the right idea."

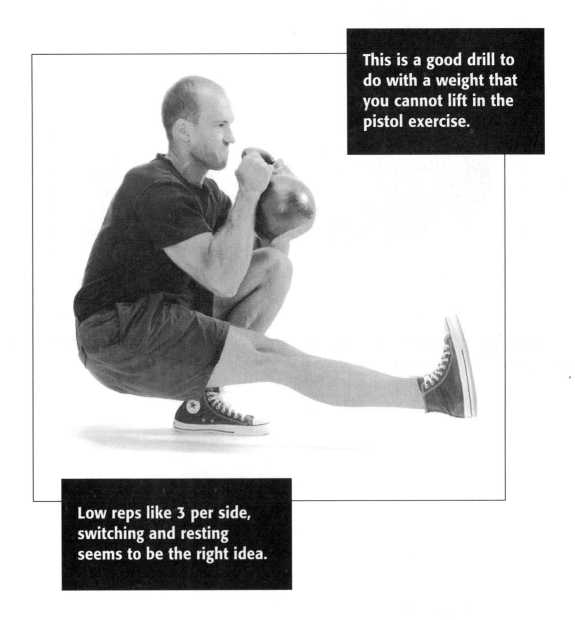

This is a good drill to do with a weight that you cannot lift in the pistol exercise.

Low reps like 3 per side, switching and resting seems to be the right idea.

Cossack Pistol

Another advanced pistol variation calls for sitting in the rock bottom position with one leg straight in front then explosively switching legs.

Keep your weight on your heel!

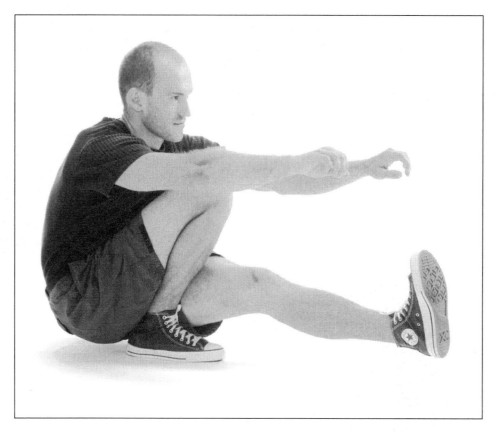

Doing this off your toes is nothing but a balance stunt; off your heels it is a power drill. Make sure to lean and reach forward for balance.

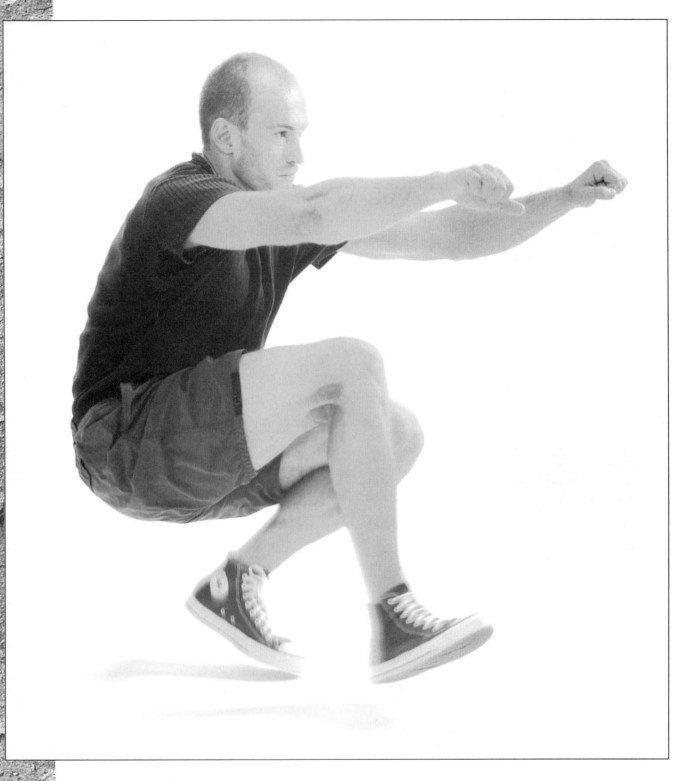

Explosively grunt as you switch feet; imagine placing a focused front heel kick into a target. Naturally, this drill is only for healthy knees and powerful legs.

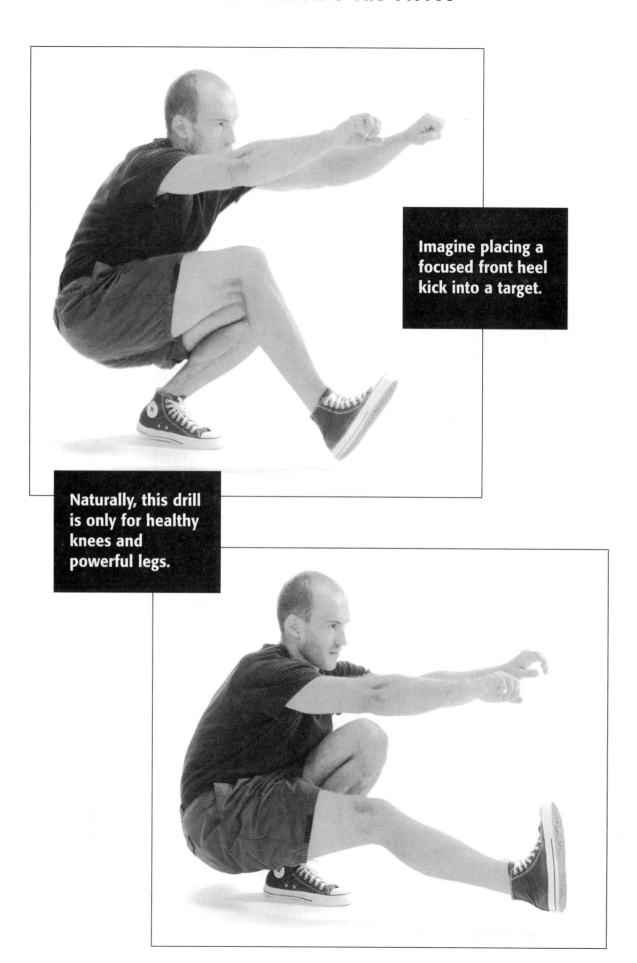

Imagine placing a focused front heel kick into a target.

Naturally, this drill is only for healthy knees and powerful legs.

Dynamic Isometric Pistol

Alright, you can knock off a dozen one-legged squats and fancy yourself to be a stud. It is time to be humbled, Comrade.

Go down rock bottom and pause there for a few seconds without relaxing.

Slowly go up until your thigh is parallel to the ground and pause again. Breathe shallow, stay tight, and enjoy the pain!

Go up another couple of inches and repeat the drill. Then finally stand up all the way. Cut in the soundtrack of evil laughter.

Combining dynamic exercise with high-tension stops at sticking points enables one to greatly increase the difficulty of strength exercise without adding weight.

Russians are better at training than marketing. They constantly invent cool techniques but often forget to name them. Such is the case with "dynamic isometrics" that owes its title to American sports scientist Dr. Michael Yessis. The essence of this powerful technique is interrupting a normal, dynamic lift with stops at certain brutal positions. The standard duration of this pause in Russia is 1-5 sec but this is not writ in stone. There can be one or more stops; always at the most difficult points of the exercise.

You could go rock bottom, go up to parallel, and pause there. For the record, most "parallel" squats you witness at gyms are a joke. The Naked Warrior defines "parallel" in powerlifting terms: the top of your knee must be above the crease on the top of your thigh.

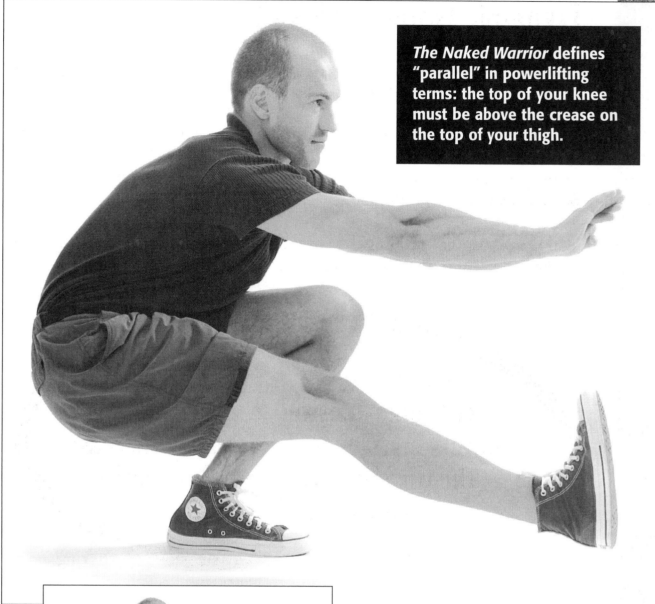

The Naked Warrior defines "parallel" in powerlifting terms: the top of your knee must be above the crease on the top of your thigh.

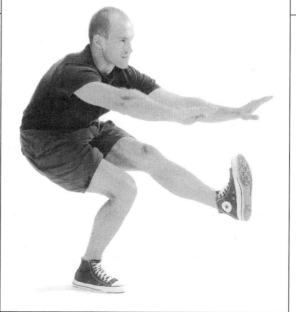

A second option is to pause an inch or two above parallel, which is a typical sticking point. Then, if you are a real hombre, stand up all the way.

141

A third option is to go rock bottom and stay there for a few seconds without relaxing, then exploding up.

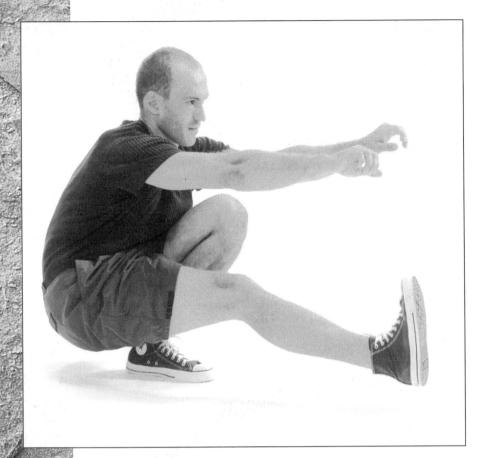

Multiple stops are truly evil. An advanced Naked Warrior can pause in the rock bottom position, then at parallel, then a couple of inches above parallel. Yes, even a very strong man can get a top quality strength workout without any equipment!

Easier variations are also possible. For instance, you could lower yourself to parallel, enjoy the pain there, and get up without going into a full squats. You may only be able to pause for a second; that is cool. Dynamic isometrics is a flexible regimen; use your imagination.

Combining dynamic exercise with high-tension stops at sticking points builds strength better than dynamic or isometric exercise alone.

In one study adding isos to dynamic lifting improved the latter's effectiveness by more than 15%! It is easy to identify at least three reasons why:

First, spending so much time under tension at the sticking point. Compare that to the usual practice of riding through using momentum.

Second, dynamic isos teach you better tension skills. You cannot help using more tension to get a dead weight moving.

Third, this type of training builds muscle.

Adding isometric stops to "normal" dynamic strength training makes it up to 15% more effective.

Dynamic isos, with a pistol variation that is easy for you, is a great way to make your knees more resistant to injury. Says pistol master Steve Cotter, RKC Sr., "be aware of any point in the range of motion that feels unstable in the knee…be more mindful in the practice (practice perfect reps) and you will be able to identify and correct any weak links in the chain." In this case we are not talking about a weak point in the range of motion but literally a weak spot around your knee.

When the goal is to make your knees more injury resistant, literally focus on the vulnerable feeling spot(s) around your knee rather that on a weak point in the range of motion.

If the doc says it is not his problem, treat these spots as "leakages". Plug them up with tension with the help of dynamic isometrics. Pick a much easier pistol variation, hold on to something for balance for extra safety, and go slow. When you have reached the weak spot, pause for a few seconds and pay attention to what it takes to generate tension there. Be mindful. Pick up the slack in the weak spot. Surround it with tension. Try to make your whole leg feel like a solid block.

Stop long before failure. Do not practice this or any other technique as self-treatment for a knee injury. This is a prevention measure for healthy knees.

After a few workouts your knees will feel a lot stronger.

Isometric Pistol

Pure isometrics are great too. The Naked Warrior does them with his characteristic efficiency. Instead of the traditional three different angles with multiple contractions at each he works just one position, the very bottom, with only one long contraction per set.

In the seventies Russian scientists Zatsiorsky and Raitsin busted the myth that isos only build strength at the specific angles they are practiced. They also learned that working just the stretched position such as the bottom of the pistol or the one-arm pushup builds strength throughout the full range of motion. That saves time, Comrade!

Later Soviet and Western research revealed a surprising fact that the intensity of the isometric contraction is not very important. But the daily time under tension is. So, "why not hold a less intense contraction up to a few minutes long?" asked sharp men of strength, such as strength coach extraordinaire Jay Schroeder and strongman author Steve Justa. Indeed.

Just stay in the rock bottom pistol position for up to a couple of minutes. Do not just sit there relaxing as you did when working on your flexibility. Push—remember the "static stomp" —steady but not too hard. Make sure to keep your hamstring tensed. Slowly build up the tension to half your max, take two to three seconds. Once more: hold it steady! If tension wavers all over the place you are wasting your time.

About half your max intensity is plenty. Be clear that 50% intensity does not refer to trying half of your best throughout the set. It means you start out with 50% of your max strength and hold it. As you get tired, you will be working harder and harder to maintain that level of force. Just like lifting a 50% 1RM weight for reps.

Release the tension just as gradually. Quit before you fail; it is important! Do not sweat it if you can hold the contraction for just a few seconds in the beginning.

Do not hold up your free leg; that would be just asking for worthless hip flexor cramps. Just rest the heel of your unloaded leg on the deck in front of you.

Although the tension is submaximal you must make an effort to use all the high-tension techniques, just powered down. Use the exact technique you use for the dynamic pistol.

Keep your abdomen compressed but do not hold your breath; breathe shallow.

Make sure to stretch the front top of your thigh afterwards; the hip flexors are easy to overwork.

**It bears repeating:
the hip flexors on the top of
your thigh cannot handle as much
volume as your quads or glutes.
You must build up your load slowly
and stretch your hip flexors
after each set.**

Isos offer many advantages and make an excellent complement to dynamic strength training.

Weighted Pistol

You may practice any of the above variations, except for the airborne lunge, with a weight held in front of you. Five or ten pounds will make it easier by improving your balance and helping you to fire your hamstrings and glutes. A heavier weight will, naturally, make it harder.

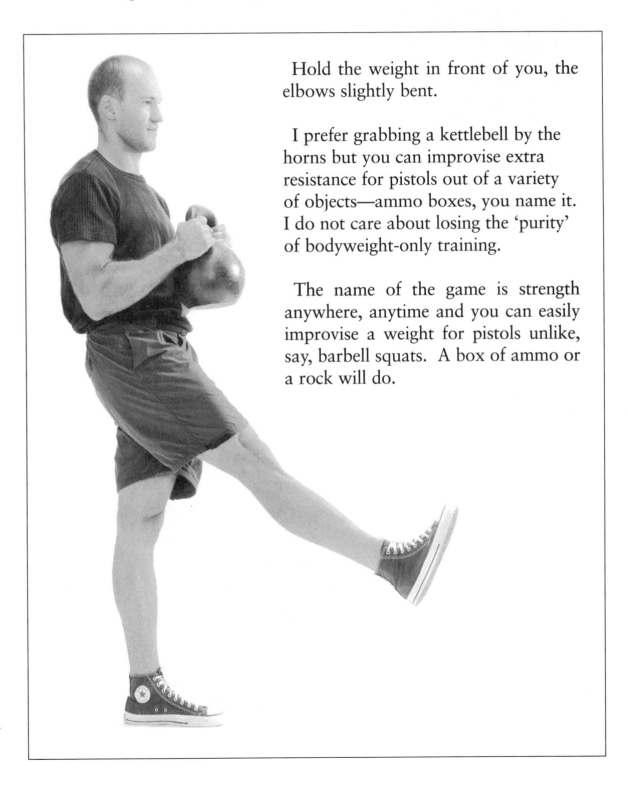

Hold the weight in front of you, the elbows slightly bent.

I prefer grabbing a kettlebell by the horns but you can improvise extra resistance for pistols out of a variety of objects—ammo boxes, you name it. I do not care about losing the 'purity' of bodyweight-only training.

The name of the game is strength anywhere, anytime and you can easily improvise a weight for pistols unlike, say, barbell squats. A box of ammo or a rock will do.

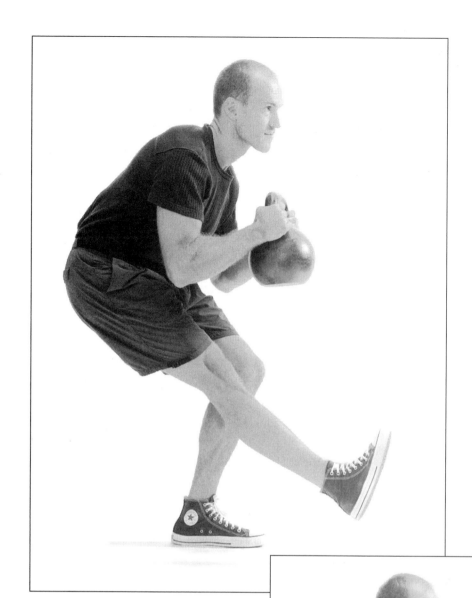

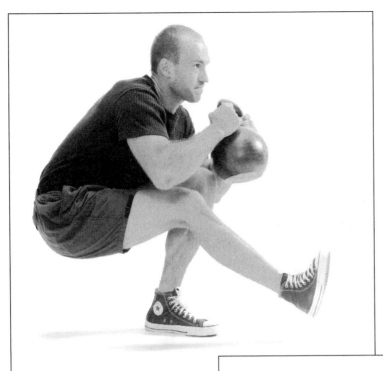

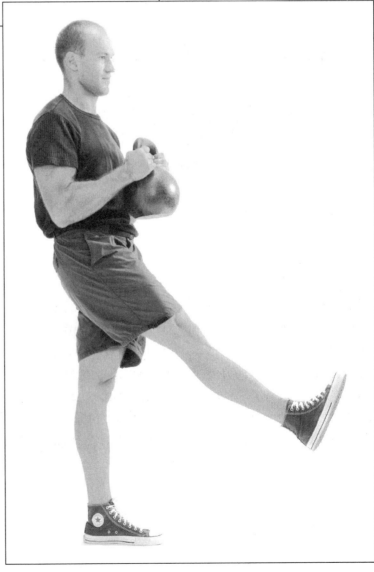

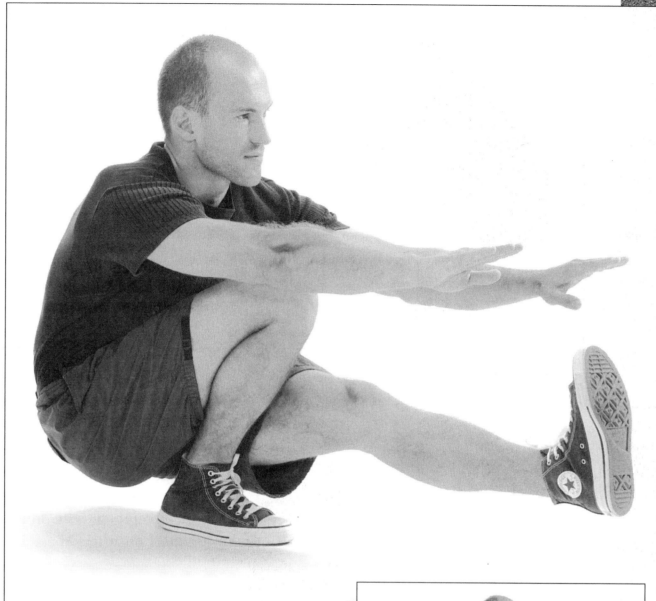

Where bodyweight pistols can be compared to relatively upright Olympic style barbell squats, heavy weighted pistols are closer to powerlifting style squats: there is more forward lean, sometimes almost as much as in the good morning. Accordingly, there is more hamstring and even lower back involvement.

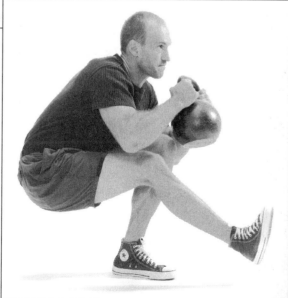

It is remarkable that you can work your spinal erectors with a relatively light weight—most Party members stick to 53 and 72 pound kettlebells. It makes sense if you think about it; holding the kettlebell way in front of you loads your back muscles because of poor leverage. This is great news, as a big downfall of bodyweight exercises is the lack of functional stress to the lower back.

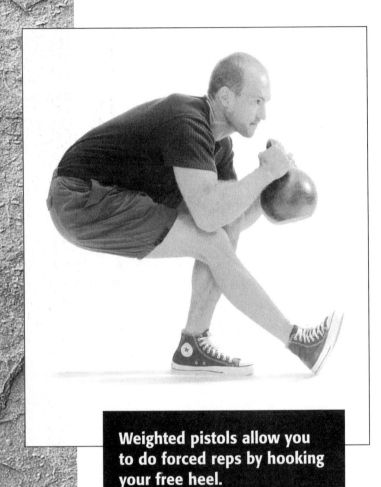

Weighted pistols allow you to do forced reps by hooking your free heel.

Note that weighted pistols allow you to do forced reps by hooking your free heel. It is not a good idea with bodyweight only pistols as this maneuver is likely to make your knee slip forward.

"I believe that Pistols are definitely one of the greatest leg strengtheners I've ever done," stated Dan 'X-celsior' Webb on the dragondoor.com forum. "I've squatted over 360 pounds in the past, but I didn't like how huge my legs were getting so I quit squatting. Doing daily Pistols (16kgx3, 24kgx3, 24kg or 32kgx3) [36, 53, and 72 pound kettlebells respectively], I feel much stronger now than I did then."

CHAPTER SEVEN

FIELD-STRIPPING THE ONE-ARM PUSHUP

- The One-Arm Pushup, Floor and Elevated
- Isometric One-Arm Pushup
- The One-Arm Dive Bomber Pushup
- The One-Arm Pump
- The One-Arm Half Bomber Pushup
- Four More Drills to Work up to the One-Arm Dive Bomber
- The One-Arm/One-Leg Pushup

The One-Arm Pushup, Floor and Elevated

If you think that once you knock off some magic number of regular pushups, say one hundred, you will automatically be able to do the one-arm pushup you have another thing coming.

The ability to carry on for a long time at a low intensity does not enable one to shine in a brief high-tension exertion. Besides, the one-arm pushup has a difficult balance element so do not expect much unless you train for it specifically.

A Catch-22, right? In order to learn how to do one-arm pushups you must do one-arm pushups, but you cannot do one-arm pushups...

Do not despair, Comrade, you can practice an easier version of the drill, with your hand on the bench, the desk, or even the wall.

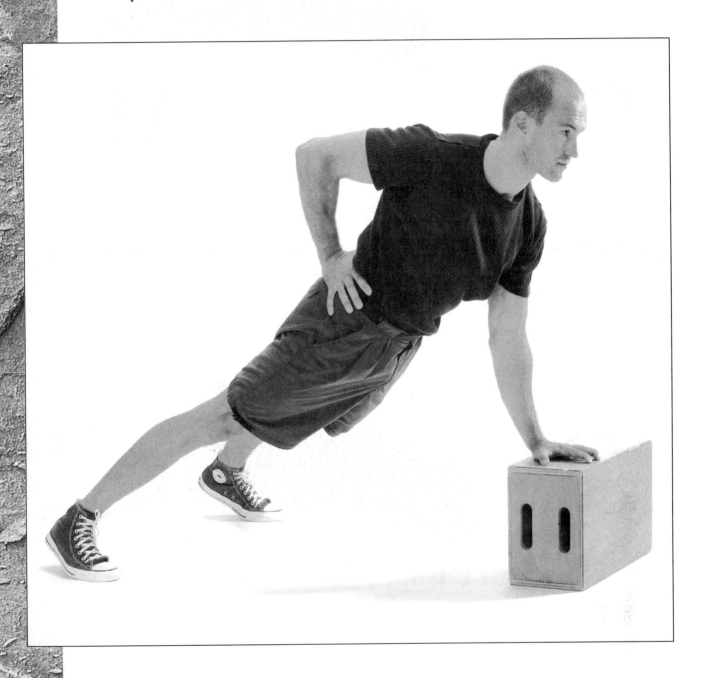

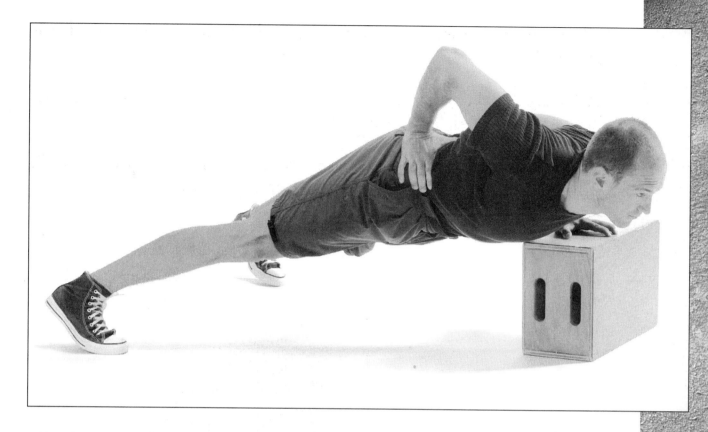

By the same token, you can make your one-armers harder by elevating your feet.

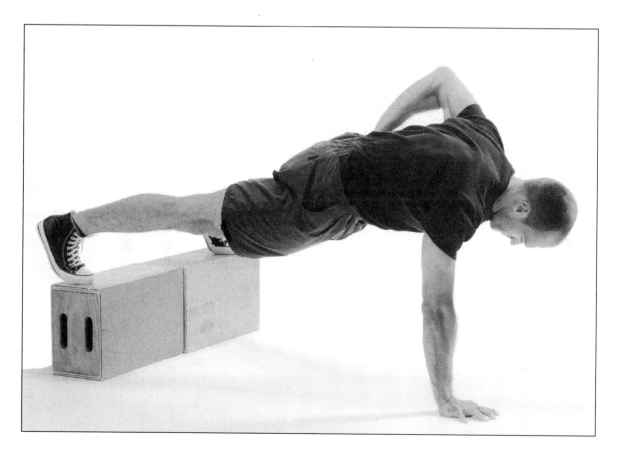

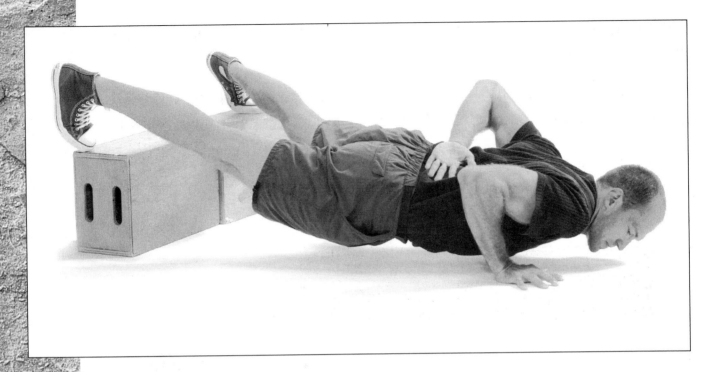

Even the one-legged version can be made harder—like it is necessary—by elevating your foot.

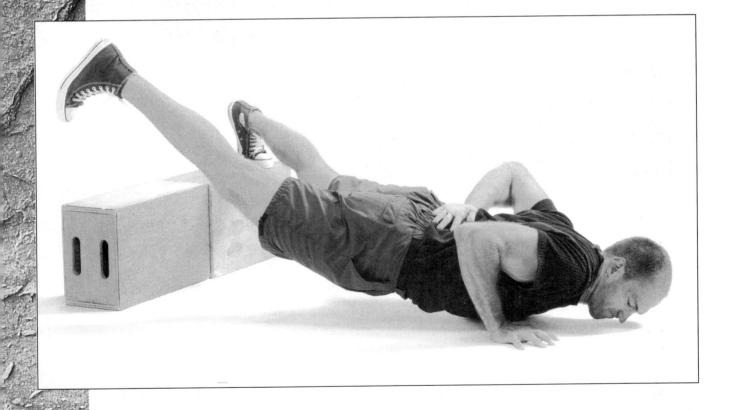

The technique of the elevated one arm pushup (either way) is identical to the floor version. Here it comes.

Let us make it clear that a legit one-arm pushup is done with the shoulders parallel to the deck, with the balls of your feet rather than their edges in contact with the surface, and all the way down until your chest almost brushes the deck.

Here is the authorized technique.

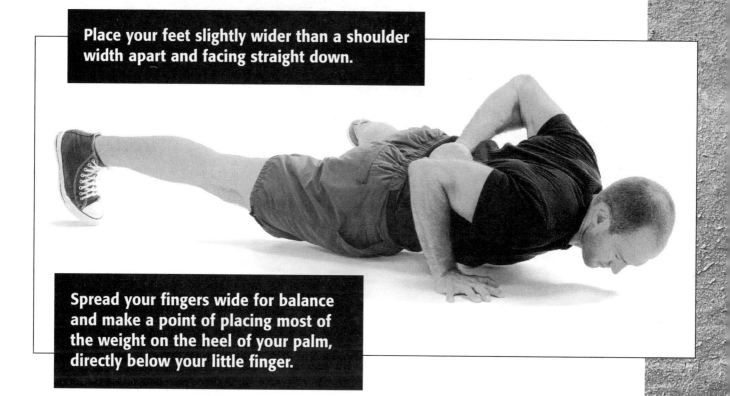

Place your feet slightly wider than a shoulder width apart and facing straight down.

Spread your fingers wide for balance and make a point of placing most of the weight on the heel of your palm, directly below your little finger.

Place your feet slightly wider than a shoulder width apart and facing straight down.

Place your working hand a couple inches outside your centerline, point your middle finger straight forward. Spread your fingers wide for balance and make a point of placing most of the weight on the heel of your palm, directly below your little finger.

Now go ahead and do a pushup. Chances are, your body will act as a disorganized "collection of body parts", your back will sag like a camel's, and the shoulder of the unloaded arm will come up first thus declaring your rep null and void.

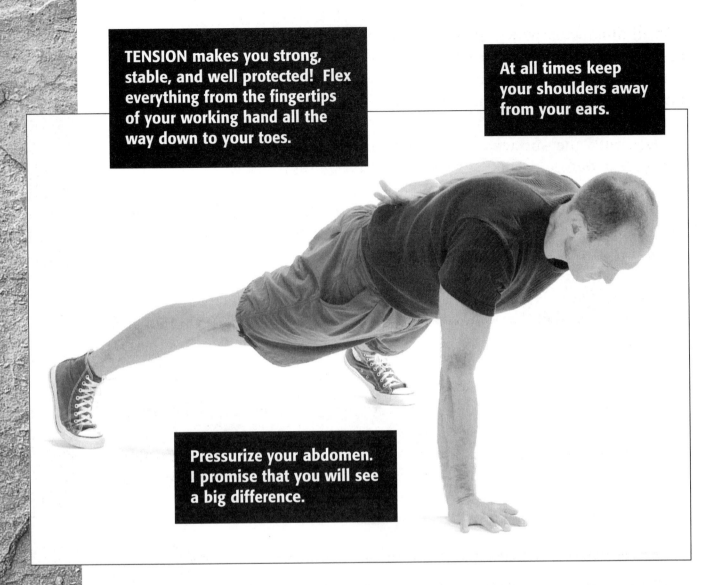

TENSION makes you strong, stable, and well protected! Flex everything from the fingertips of your working hand all the way down to your toes.

At all times keep your shoulders away from your ears.

Pressurize your abdomen. I promise that you will see a big difference.

Rewind and start all over. First, brace your whole body before lowering your chest to the deck, bench, or wall. Do not ever forget that it is TENSION that makes you strong, stable, and well protected! Flex everything from the fingertips of your working hand all the way down to your toes.

Nice and tight, lower your chest to the deck or the bench. Chances are, you will either collapse before you hit the bottom or your body will get so crooked that innocent bystanders might think you are practicing yoga.

Here is how to develop a crisp and controlled descent:

Instead of yielding to your weight with your triceps, push your chest out and actively pull yourself to the ground with your lat. That is right, like in a one-arm row. You will be amazed how much easier it is to do things the evil Russian way and how your shoulder immediately stops protesting.

At all times keep your shoulders away from your ears. Apply a corkscrew action to the ground. Do not simply keep your elbow close to your ribs; actively, externally rotate the shoulder, "screw" your arm into the floor from inside out. Do it on the way down and even more on the way up.

Pressurize your abdomen. I promise that you will see a big difference. Naturally, your quads and cheeks must also stay tight.

Make sure that your shoulders stay parallel to the deck for the duration of the set; leading with your unloaded shoulder does not qualify and is a poor workout.

As you get stronger, start lowering your bench until your hand is on the floor and you are doing a legit one-arm pushup. Then you can take on this drill with your feet elevated, first a couple of inches off the floor and then higher and higher.

You can make the one-arm pushup tougher without elevating your feet by throwing a chain or a sandbag on top of your neck. No chain? Then try a bag with barbell plates wrapped in a towel. Not only is this more comfortable than carrying it on your back, the pressure on your neck extensors will add juice to your triceps and upper back muscles.

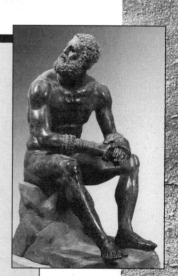

ARE YOUR WRISTS GIVING YOU TROUBLE AFTER PUSHUPS AND SIMILAR DRILLS?

Provided there are no medical issues you can reduce the discomfort with a counter stretch between sets. Kneel on a reasonably soft surface such as grass, a mat, or a carpet. Flex your wrists, lock out your elbows, and place your hands on the deck, the palms up and the fingers facing back. Carefully lean forward and stretch your wrists for five seconds. Repeat for a couple of sets.

Continued next page.

As your ligaments get stronger you may try your pushups in that position, "pushups on fins", as we called them in Spetsnaz. As an option, the fingers may point in towards each other. Strive to get a complete elbow extension. Build up slow!

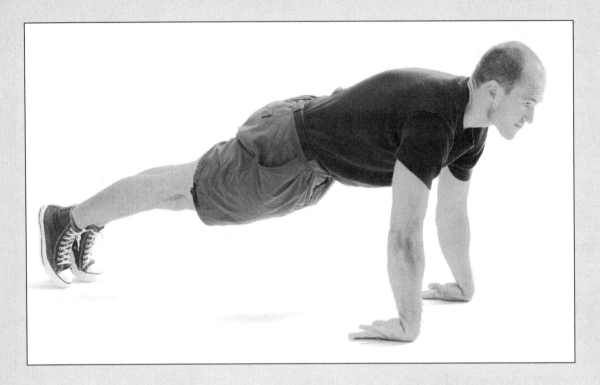

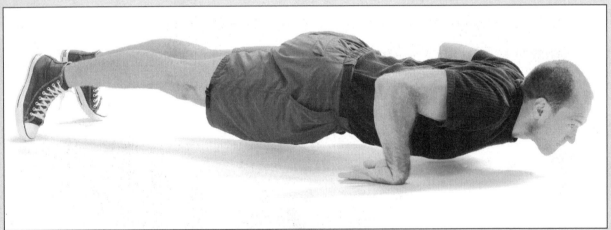

If your wrists just cannot handle the hyperextension imposed on them by regular pushups, here is a different course of action:

Switch to pushups on your fists. They will force your wrists to get stronger without overstretching. At the same time the whole exercise will be harder, thanks to an extended range of motion. Harder and safer. The Party way.

In the martial arts tradition do your fist pushups on the first and second knuckles on horizontal fists; the second and the third knuckles on vertical fists. In the beginning using the whole surface of the fist is OK. Work up slowly; don't let your wrists buckle on you.

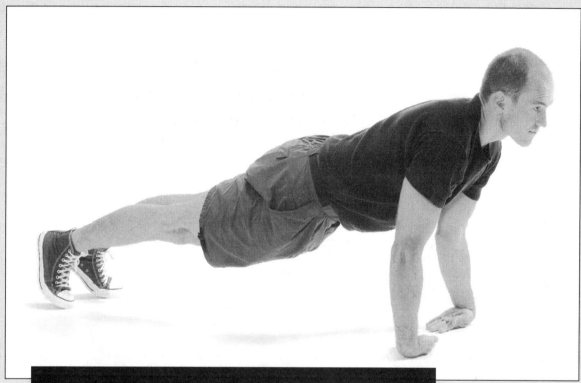

Pause for a few seconds and staying tight at the sticking points of the exercise before moving along.

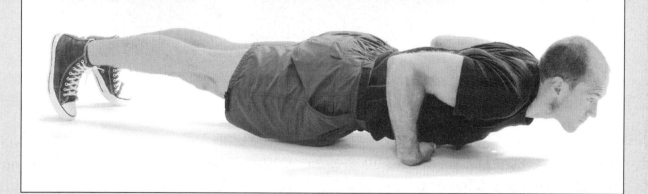

Isometric One-Arm Pushup

Gymnasts and rock climbers boast outstanding pound per pound strength. One of their secrets is combining dynamic and static strength training. Leonid Lapshin, one of Russia's top mountain men, the first in the USSR to earn the Master of Sports ranking in both mountaineering and rock climbing, recommends the 70 to 30 ratio of dynamic and static strength training.

Lie on your stomach, tense all over, and push. Even though your body will not clear the deck make a point of keeping your legs and waist rigid. Your body should feel lighter, like it is almost ready to take off.

You might prefer working these with your hand up on an elevation, even a wall. In that case keep your chest airborne. Advanced Naked Warriors can stay off the deck even in floor one-armers.

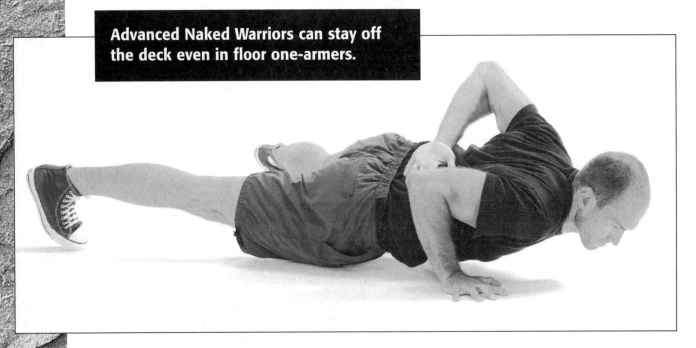

Advanced Naked Warriors can stay off the deck even in floor one-armers.

Breathe shallow, stay tight and work on your mind-to-muscle connection. Look for "leakages" and weak spots and plug them up with tension; pick out the slack. Your body should feel like one rigid block. This strength skill enhancement is one of the many benefits of isometrics.

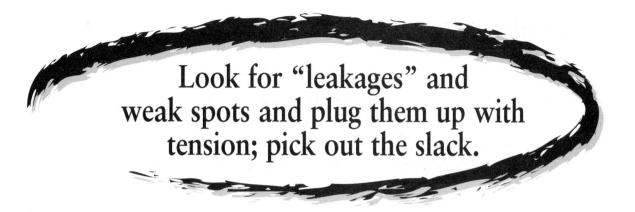

Look for "leakages" and
weak spots and plug them up with
tension; pick out the slack.

Employ a long, steady, submaximal tension; the same drill as with the iso
pistol. Take your time working up to a minute and more; it is okay to start
with seconds.

The One-Arm Dive Bomber Pushup

To do this evil variation of the Navy SEAL favorite you need to descend at
an angle rather than straight down, squeeze under an imaginary fence, and
end up in the one arm cobra.

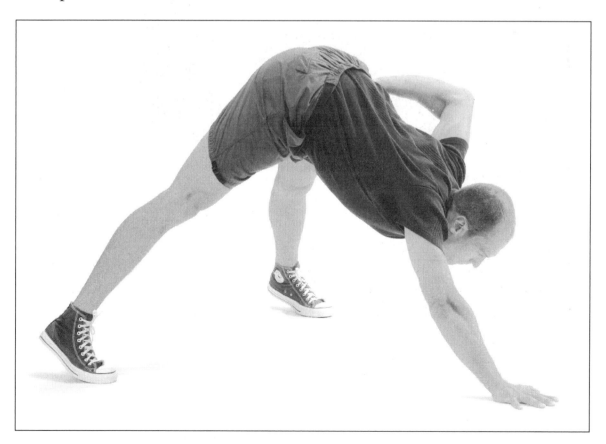

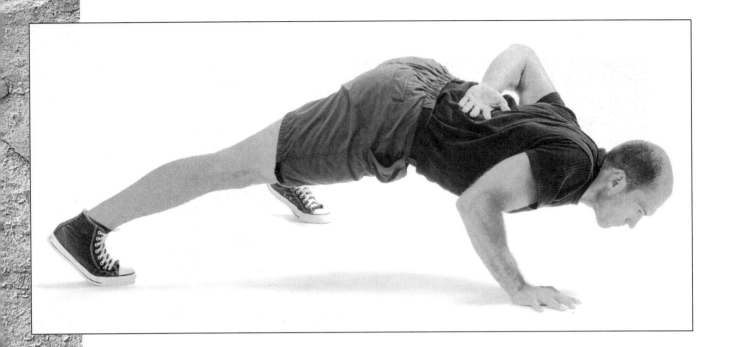

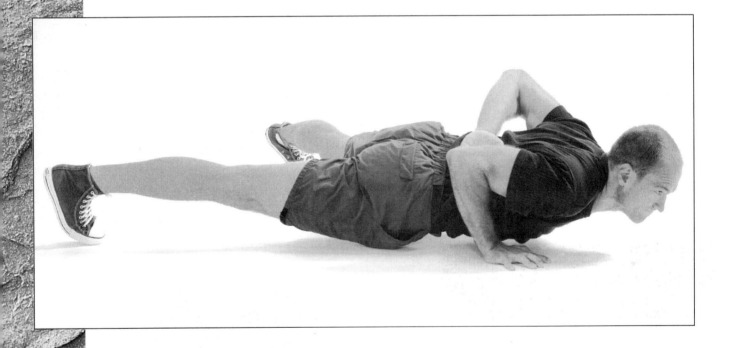

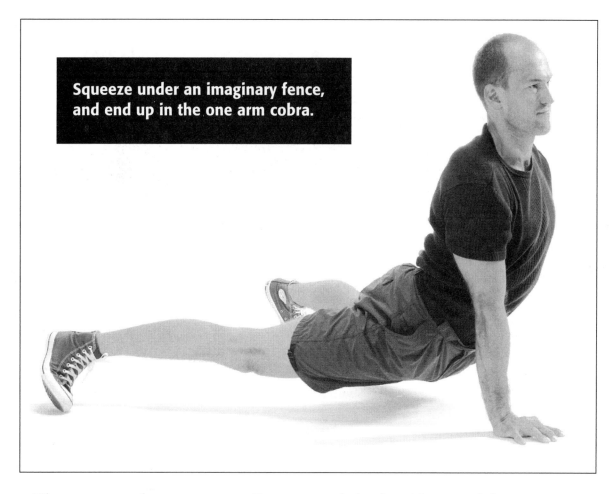

Squeeze under an imaginary fence, and end up in the one arm cobra.

Then reverse the movement. Do not push back with a straight arm as you would in a Hindu pushup; go back under the fence! This exercise is easy to cheat on by cutting depth and not moving in an arc—don't!

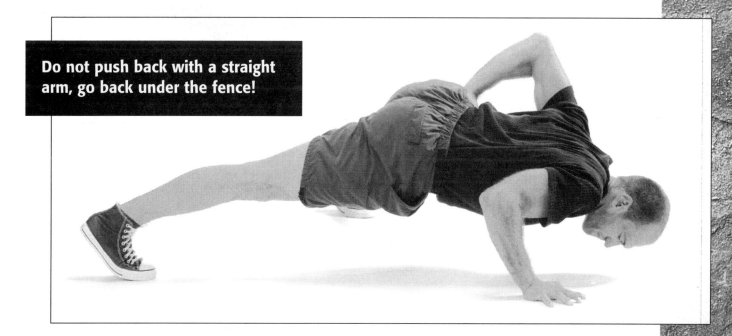

Do not push back with a straight arm, go back under the fence!

Steve Maxwell, RKC Sr., suggested this great imagery: as you are going down think of a negative military press; when you are worming under and up pretend that you are doing a triceps cable pushdown. On the way back it is the "military press from your stomach".

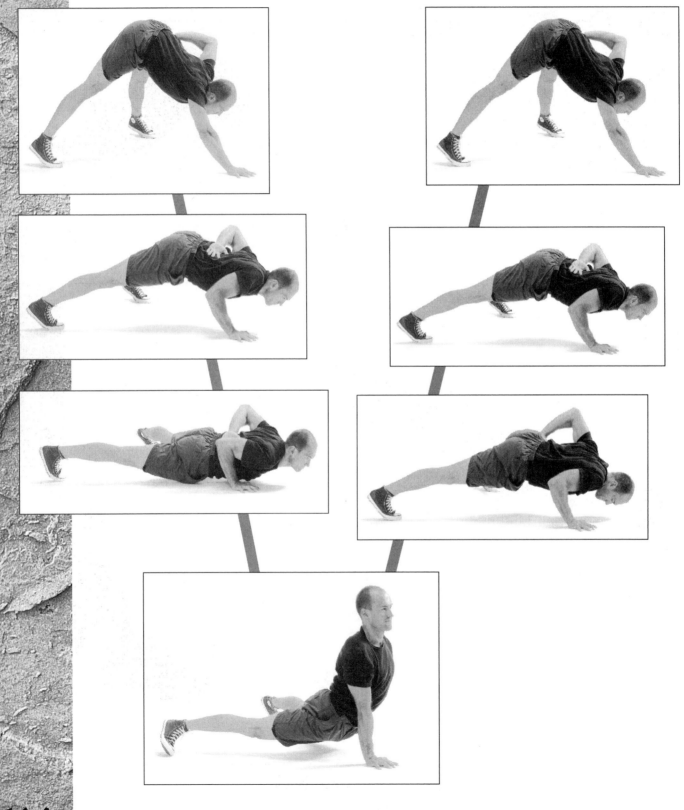

I bet evergreen dollars against Russian roubles that you will fail at first. You need a sound progression strategy. Here it is.

The One-Arm Pump

Plant your hand, the fingers spread wide, approximately in line with your shoulder and the other behind your back. Keep your arm straight and go from...

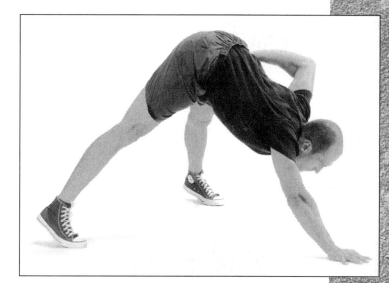

...through...

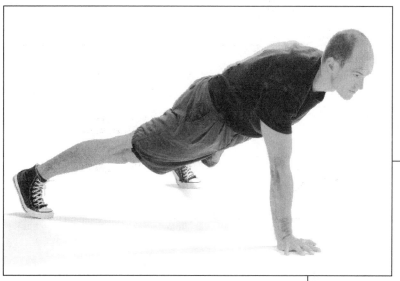

...to...

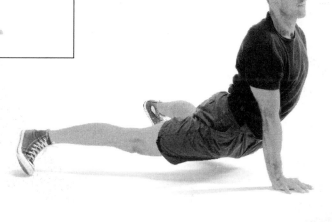

...and back.

This drill is known as "prokachka"—roughly translated as "the pump" in Russian—and will teach you the proper balance for the one-arm dive bomber.

Pull down with your lat; push back up with your deltoid while keeping your armpit tight.

Do not be afraid to move your feet or hand to find the optimal position.

The One-Arm Half Bomber Pushup

From the standard jackknifed position descend at an angle like a landing bomber until your chest almost brushes the deck and your elbow is fully flexed and tucked into your side.

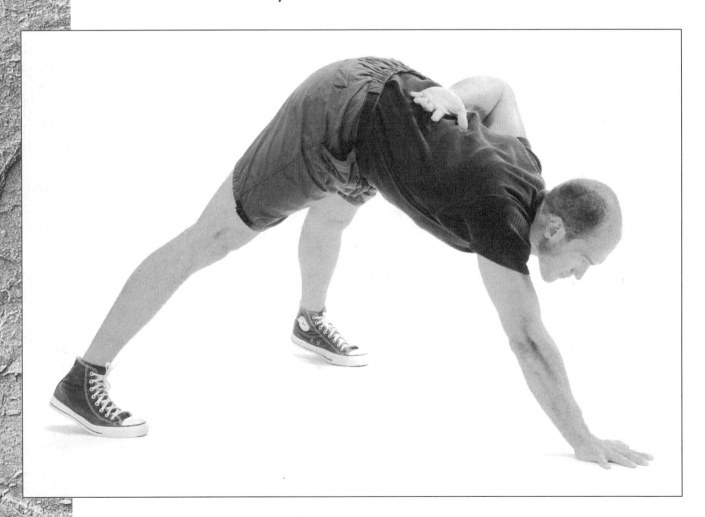

Or at least almost there.

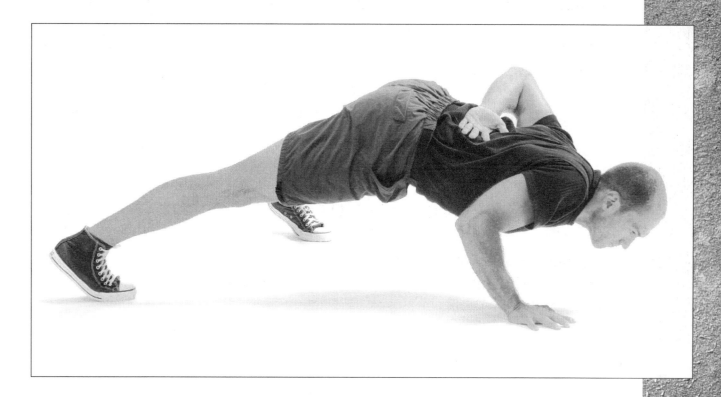

Push back, again at an angle rather than straight up. The groove is identical to that of the military press.

Some tips on keeping you safe. Do not take a ridiculously wide stance and do not let your ankles pronate or buckle in—which is the easy thing to do. You will be on your toes but your ankles should be almost perpendicular to the deck. Ask your chiropractor why this is so important.

It is imperative that you keep your shoulder pushed away from your ear and pushed back!

It is imperative that your elbow stays very close to your body; come to think of it, the exercise is not possible otherwise.

The active negative plus the corkscrew will take care of both.

Four More Drills
to Work up to the One-Arm Dive Bomber

Working your way back "under the fence" will be hard, very hard.

Two-arm/one-leg dive-bombers will help.

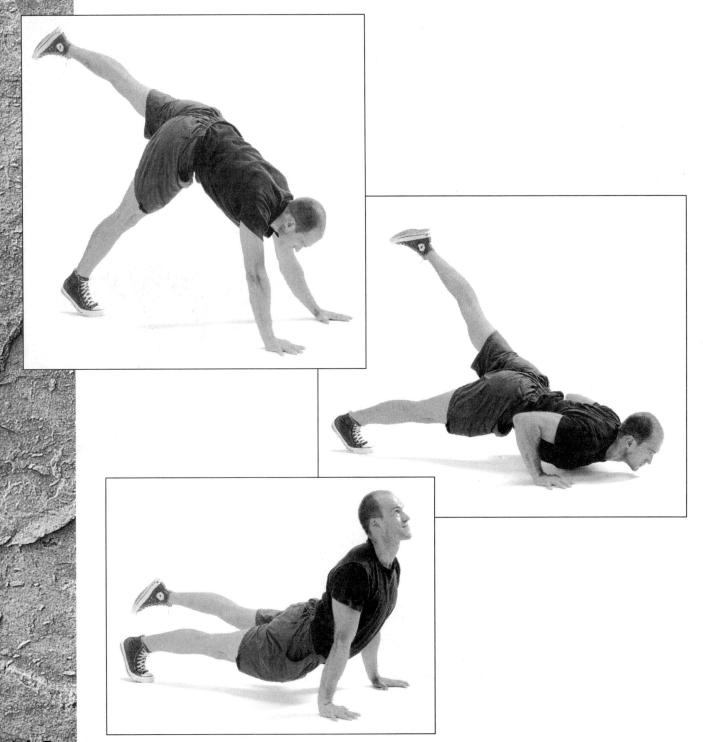

So will dive-bombers with your free palm placed on top of the hand of the working arm and helping some.

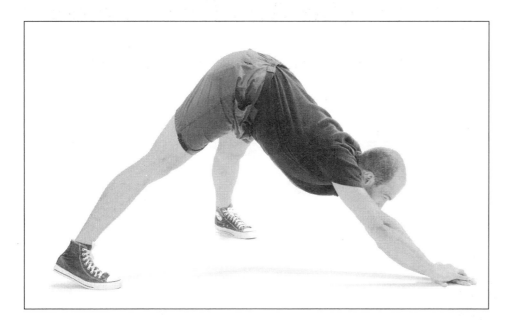

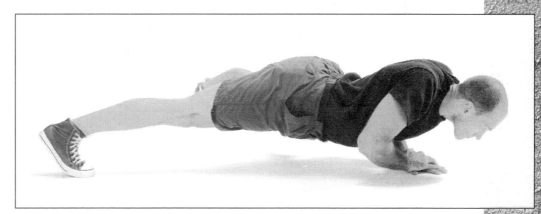

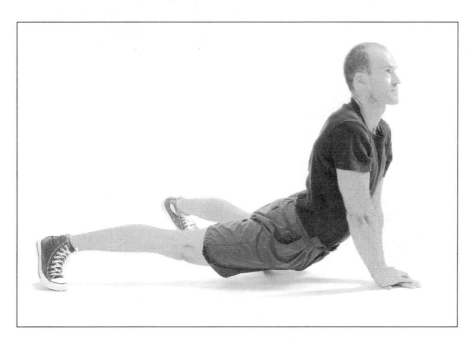

Another good assistance exercise is a partial (a few inches) two-arm dive-bomber through the sticking point at the bottom of the arc.

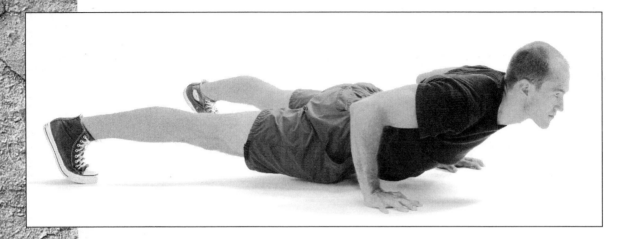

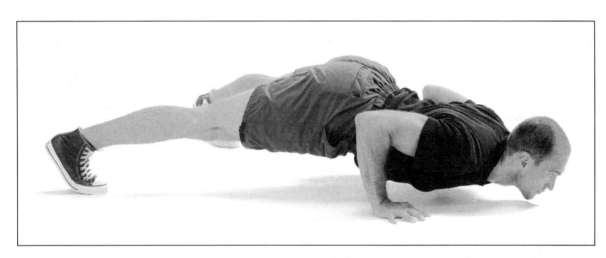

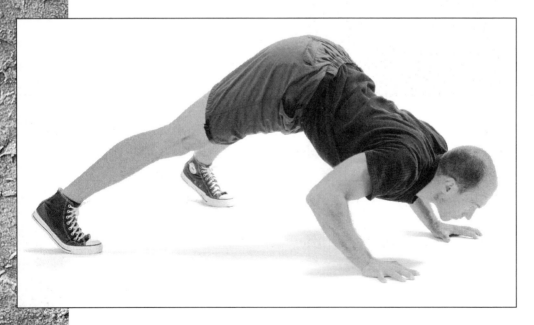

Remember to keep your shoulders screwed into their sockets. Think "triceps pushdown" as you go forward and "military press" on the way back.

The One-Arm/One-Leg Pushup

Finally, the Tsar of the one-arm pushups:

The instructions are identical to those for the regular one arm pushup, with two additional tips.

First, get yourself tight and rock solid and find your balance by moving your planted hand and foot and your free leg.

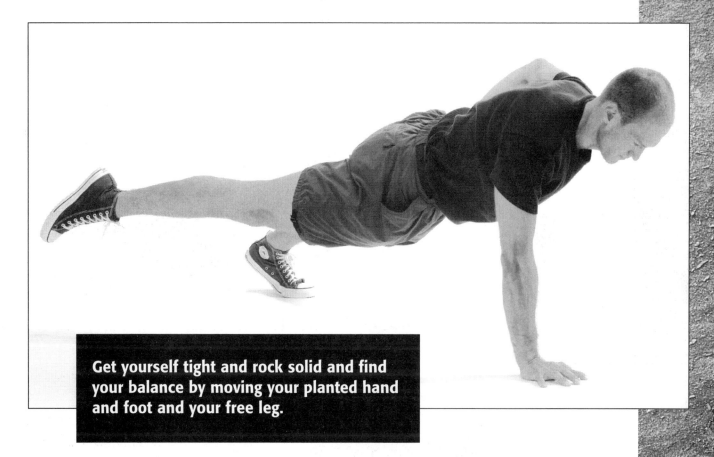

Get yourself tight and rock solid and find your balance by moving your planted hand and foot and your free leg.

Unless you brace your whole body and form a tight "power line" from the toes of your left foot through your rock hard stomach, through your flexed right lat, and all the way into the fingertips of your right hand, you will topple like the Taliban. Keep practicing the tension and you will get the hang of it.

Do not even think of resting your weight on the edge of your foot—that is cheating!

Once more, throughout the pushup keep your pushing hand, your planted foot, and your lower abdomen rigidly in line. To quote Masatoshi Nakayama again, "Tensing the muscles on the front and sides of the abdomen links the pelvis and the shoulders. A stable pelvis and the complementary muscle groups of the thigh working together contribute to strong movements and a stable stance. This strong foundation gives support and makes it possible for the power of the hips to be transmitted to the arm."

Enjoy the pain!

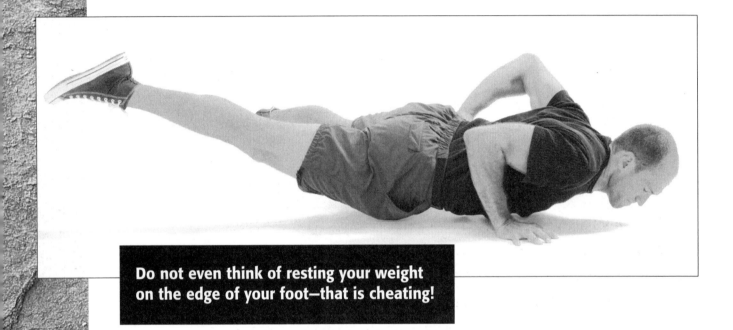

Do not even think of resting your weight on the edge of your foot—that is cheating!

CHAPTER EIGHT

NAKED WARRIOR Q&A

- Are bodyweight exercises superior to exercises with weights?
- Why is there such an intense argument in the martial arts community as to whether bodyweight exercises are superior to exercises with weights?
- Can I get very strong using only bodyweight exercises?
- Should I mix different strength-training tools in my training?
- How can I incorporate bodyweight exercises with kettlebell and barbell training?
- Can the high-tension techniques and GTG system be applied to weights?
- Can the high-tension techniques and GTG system be applied to strength endurance training?
- I can't help overtraining. What should I do?
- Can I follow the Naked Warrior program on an ongoing basis?
- Can I add more exercises to the Naked Warrior program?
- Will my development be unbalanced from doing only two exercises?
- Is there a way to work the lats with a pulling exercise when no weights or pullup bars are accessible?
- How should I apply the Naked Warrior techniques to my sport-specific conditioning?

- Where can I learn more about bodyweight-only strength training?
- Low reps and no failure? This training is too easy!
- Will I forget it all the strength techniques in some sort of emergency?
- Isn't dedicating most of the book to technique too much?
- Power to you, Naked Warrior!

Are bodyweight exercises superior to exercises with weights?

Neither is superior. Various types of resistance have advantages and disadvantages. Here is how the most common ones stack up against each other.

Bodyweight

The calisthenics' advantage is their accessibility, first and foremost. I could give you a non-scientific pitch about the naturalness of calisthenics or a pseudo-scientific one about open and closed kinetic chains, but I won't. The primary advantage of bodyweight strength exercises is the fact that you can practice them anywhere and anytime.

Cals enforce a functional bodyweight and a healthy body composition. You could eat yourself into a heart attack yet excel in the bench press. That won't happen with one-arm pushups. You can't have a high ratio of strength to bodyweight if you are a fat blob (or a muscle-bound blob, for that matter).

The biggest disadvantage of bodyweight exercising is that this approach doesn't enable you to perform full-body pulling movements, such as the deadlift, the snatch, or the clean. Such moves are fundamental to training in most sports. While you could develop the muscles of the posterior chain with back bridges, back extensions, and reverse hypers, training the muscles and training the movement are "two big differences," as they say in the Russian hard town of Odessa.

The authoritative Russian *Boxing Yearbook* recommends doing explosive snatches with a weight equal to the boxer's bodyweight. Frank Shamrock said it all in his interview with Mike Mahler, RKC Sr.: "What the clean does is it builds explosiveness from your toes up and that's really where we're starting from in MMA [mixed martial arts]. Everything starts from the toes and extends to the point of the hands. It's more of a continuity thing; if you can get your body to go rip and blow that energy up, you can focus that energy in other places. Your body will remember that and be strong through that motion. It's very similar to punching."

Barbells

A barbell enables you to lift very heavy, which is just plain fun. There is nothing like the rush of locking out a bar-bending deadlift.

Apart from the testosterone bull, a true advantage of the barbell is the precisely calibrated resistance. You can easily specify something like "82.5% 1RM." Why is that important? Because it enables you to do a *power cycle*: a multiweek program that specifies exact training poundages and culminates with a strength PR. Such a cycle is very easy to implement and highly effective.

Cycling will not work with other traditional types of resistance the way it will work with barbells. Dumbbells, even if they progress in 5-lb. increments, don't allow such precision (an increase from 20 to 25 pounds is a 25 percent jump!), and kettlebells were purposefully designed to make major jumps in weight. Finally, bodyweight drills don't let you change your leverage with barbell-like precision, either.

Dumbbells

A dumbbell adds a stabilization challenge and works you more equally on both sides than a barbell. The disadvantage of using dumbbells is that you need a ton of them, which consumes cash and space. Adjustable plate-loaded dumbbells are an option. Make sure you get them from a reputable company, such as ironmind.com. You don't want them to fall apart and crack your skull!

Dumbbells are not practical for some valuable exercises. For instance, a strong trainee will have a hard time getting a quality leg workout with dumbbells. They don't get nearly heavy enough for deadlifts, they cannot be racked for front squats, and they cannot be comfortably held for pistols.

Kettlebells

I have yet to meet a hard man who has lifted a Russian kettlebell and not come away convinced that it's the ultimate in strength and conditioning. Dr. Dennis Koslowski, DC, RKC, Olympic silver medalist in Greco-Roman wrestling, flat out stated, "Kettlebells are like weightlifting times ten...If I could've met Pavel in the early '80s, I might've won two gold medals. I'm serious."

The kettlebell's design, namely a thick handle removed from a compact center of mass, is responsible for its many unique benefits. A thick and smooth handle, combined with the ballistic nature of many exercises, forges an iron grip and wrist. Last but not least on the kettlebell forearm killer list are bottom up cleans and similar drills. Offset center of gravity maximizes shoulder strength, health, and flexibility.

The position of the handle also allows dynamic passing of the kettlebell from hand to hand for a great variety of powerful juggling-type exercises, which are strongly endorsed by the Russian Federation State Committee on Physical Culture. These drills develop dynamic strength and injury-proof the body in many planes, unlike conventional linear exercises.

Another benefit of kettlebell training is that there is no need to have adjustable or numerous weights. It has evolved to provide progressive overload through other means. To use the squat as an example, you can back squat holding a kettlebell by its "horns" between your shoulder blades (which cannot be done with a dumbbell), then work up to holding it on your chest (front squats are impossible with dumbbells and can be brutal on the wrists with barbells), proceed to the Hack squats with the kettlebell held in the small of your back (again, cannot be done with a dumbbell), and then to a one-legged squat with the kettlebell held in the front by the "horns." Finally, an extremely strong comrade can do one-legged front squats with a kettlebell racked.

Thus, a single kettlebell provides an uncompromising means of developing leg strength—without the need for expensive and space-consuming barbells and squat racks. Thus, kettlebells have been called "the low-tech/high-concept strength solution for spec ops."

Being a kettlebell lifter, instructor, and businessman, I could go on forever. But you should have the idea by now: The Russian kettlebell is "a workout with balls."

I'm not going to review all the types of resistance equipment on the market. You get the idea.

One parting thought: Your sport's specificity might dictate your primary choice of type of resistance. For instance, a gymnast must emphasize bodyweight training, and a powerlifter must lift a barbell.

Why is there such an intense argument in the martial arts community as to whether bodyweight exercises are superior to exercises with weights?

Because the issue of what provides the resistance is confused with the workout design: sets, reps, rest periods, tempo, etc.

Under the terms of this pointless argument powerlifting and high rep triceps kickbacks with a Barbie dumbbell fall under the same misleading category of "weight training." The label "bodyweight training" is just as misleading, considering that one-legged squats with a one-second pause on the bottom and Hindu squats have totally different effects on your body. Apples and oranges. The pistols' effect is a lot closer to that of barbell squats—heavy, low rep barbell squats, to be exact—than to that of high-rep Hindu squats.

The point is, don't get hung up on what provides the resistance. Focus on the attribute you are trying to develop. And a fighter, unlike a weightlifter or a distance runner, needs a mix of different types of strength and endurance.

If you see a powerlifter who sucks wind on the mat or in the ring, it doesn't mean that barbells or heavy training are inappropriate for a fighter. They are simply one piece of the S&C puzzle (and he has neglected the other pieces, be it one or more subtypes of strength, endurance, skill, etc. Yakov Zobnin from Siberia, the heavyweight world champion in Kyokushinkai, "the World's Strongest Karate," squats almost 500 pounds deep enough to get white lights in any powerlifting meet, in spite of his basketball height. But he also maxes out at 25 strict pullups and practices explosive pushups, etc.

177

The bottom line. The argument about whether iron or bodyweight rules is a waste of bad breath. What you need to do is identify the different types of strength required in your style and then develop them with the types of resistance available to you. Practice low-rep, high-tension, max-strength training as outlined in *The Naked Warrior* or *Power to the People!* Do explosive drills. And don't forget your endurance. In case you didn't know, *The Russian Kettlebell Challenge* covers the complete martial arts strength and conditioning package. Just add skills and kick butt!

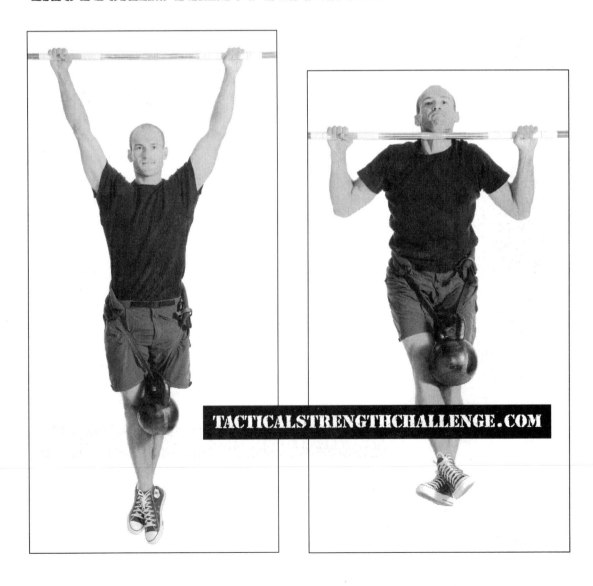

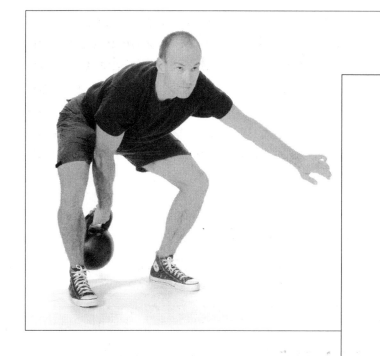

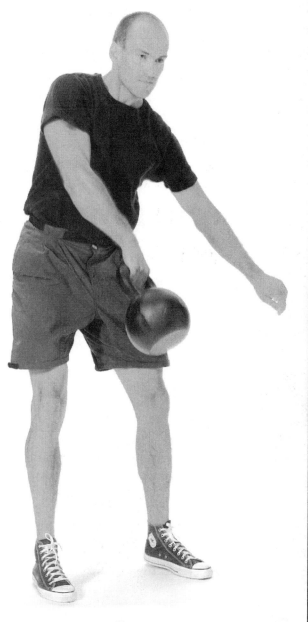

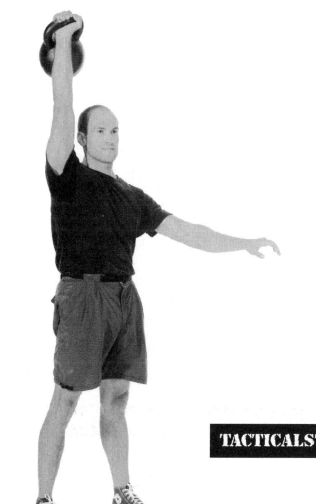

TACTICALSTRENGTHCHALLENGE.COM

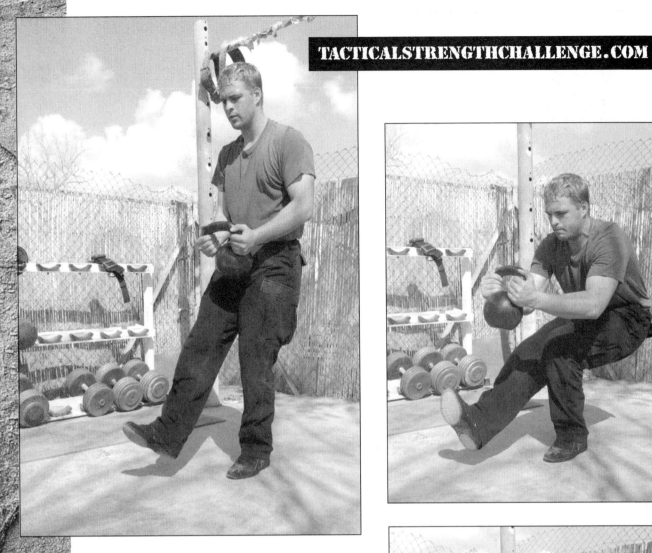

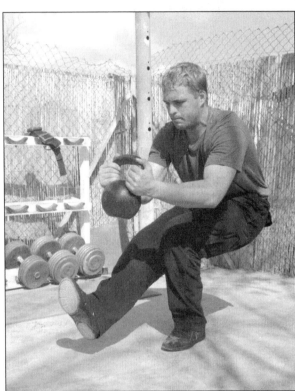

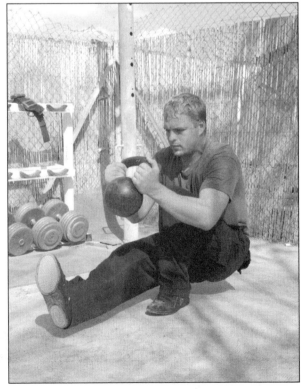

SSgt. Nate Morrison is the combatives course project manager for USAF pararescue. This Senior RKC instructor has taken his kettlebells on a "world tour" with his elite unit.. Photo courtesy Nate Morrison.

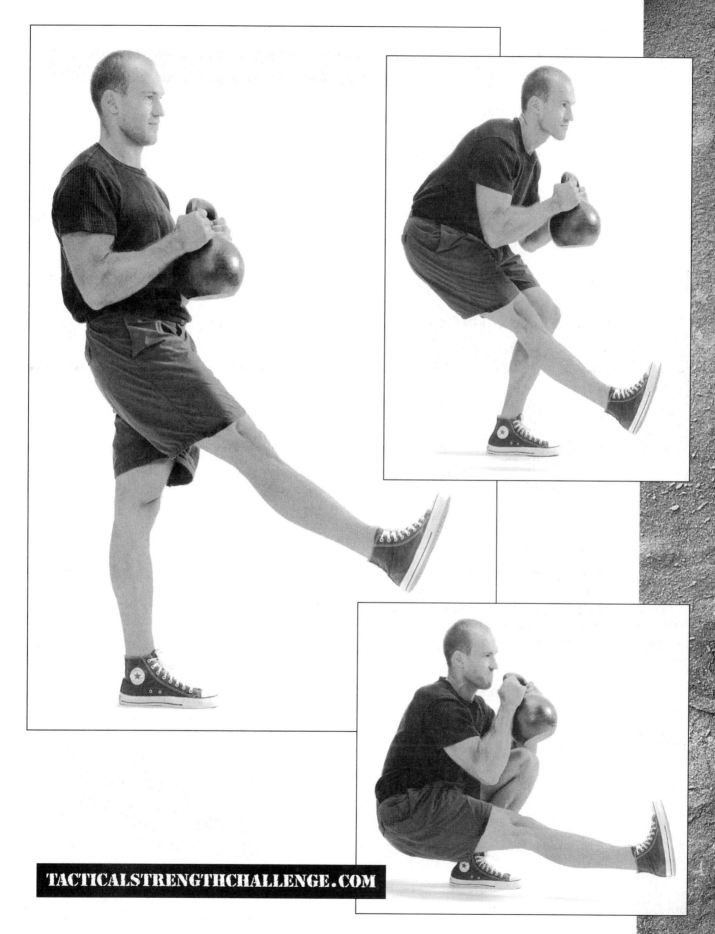

TACTICALSTRENGTHCHALLENGE.COM

Can I get very strong using only bodyweight exercises?

It depends on what you mean by 'strong'. If your goal is to become a pullup master or to achieve a planche, then yes, it can be done with bodyweight-only exercises (although using extra resistance would speed up the process). If your goal is to compete in weightlifting, then the answer is no. For martial arts, try a mix of cals with kettlebell drills.

Should I mix different strength-training tools in my training?

Ethan Reeve, RKC, the head strength and conditioning coach at Wake Forest University in North Carolina, makes great use of bodyweight, kettlebells, barbells, and many other strength tools with his athletes. So yes, you can mix different strength-training tools in your training.

The real question is, do you have Coach Reeve's knowledge and experience? No, you don't. And even if you did, you wouldn't likely have regular access to a training facility that has all those things. That reframes the issue entirely, doesn't it?

The fewer parts your training has, the less likely it is to break down. Think like Kalashnikov, the inventor of the AK-47. It's a simple, straightforward piece of equipment, but it gets the job done (and then some).

There's a reason so many hard men, like Jeff Martone and Mike Mahler stick to kettlebells and select power cals. If you are training to fight, whether in the ring or at war, they are all you need.

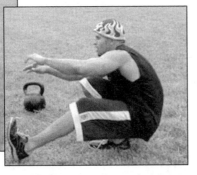

Mike Mahler RKC Sr., is a strength coach to MMA fighters and a well known strength writer. Photo courtesy *mikemahler.com*

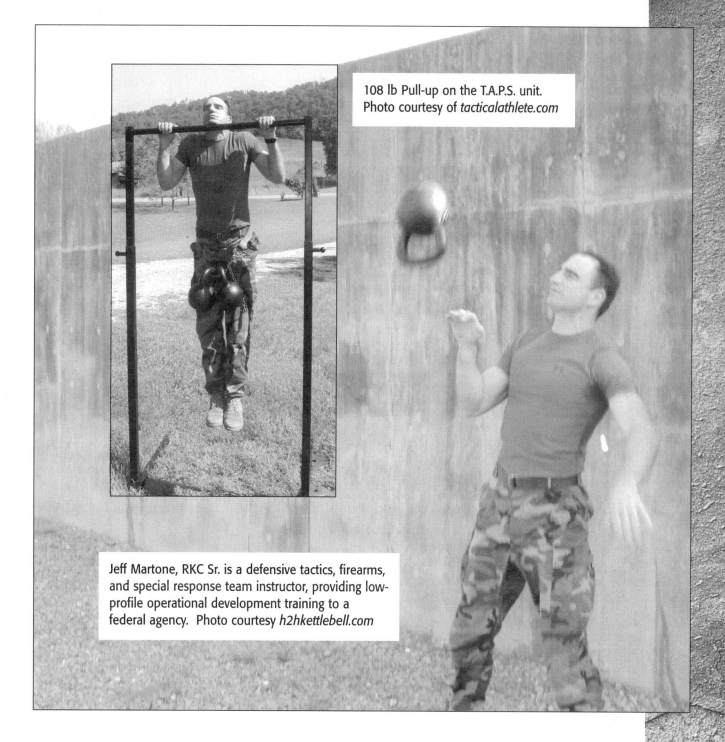

108 lb Pull-up on the T.A.P.S. unit.
Photo courtesy of *tacticalathlete.com*

Jeff Martone, RKC Sr. is a defensive tactics, firearms, and special response team instructor, providing low-profile operational development training to a federal agency. Photo courtesy *h2hkettlebell.com*

How can I incorporate bodyweight exercises with kettlebell and barbell training?

Again, don't think in terms of type of *resistance*. Think about the type of strength you want to work on.

For instance, clapping pushups, low-rep kettlebell snatches and throws, and barbell power cleans are all explosive-strength-type moves and should be done together. One-arm pushups, deadlifts, and bottom-up kettlebell clean-and-presses are all max-strength moves. Finally, repetition pushups, kettlebell snatches, and 20-rep barbell squats are strength-endurance moves.

Group your drills accordingly. The rule of thumb is to progress from explosive to max-strength drills to high reps, be it within one workout or across an entire week's training.

Can the high-tension techniques and GTG system be applied to weights?

You bet! High-tension techniques work in all sorts of high-force applications.

Ditto for the GTG, if you have access to weights throughout the day. Unless you are a gym employee, a welfare case, or a trust-fund baby, that's unlikely. You could bring your kettlebell to work, though, and add snatches to the pistol-plus-one-arm-pushup mix.

Can the high-tension techniques and GTG system be applied to strength endurance training?

Yes. Use approximately half of your max reps when "greasing" your endurance groove, and save the HTT for the last reps of your test.

I can't help overtraining. What should I do?

GTG every other day. Another option is to train for a few days in a row and then take a day off when fatigue starts setting in.

Can I follow the Naked Warrior program on an ongoing basis?

Yes, but you had better add a big pull, such as the barbell deadlift, the clean, or the kettlebell snatch. None of these has to be done daily in the GTG format. You can train it independently with a more conventional workout, say, twice a week for 5x5.

To give you an idea of what full time Naked Warrior training can do for you, here is a story of Zak Maxwell told by his BJJ world champion father:

"It probably seemed like magic to the other kids in school, when my son, Zak knocked off 16 pull-ups for a 7th grade fitness test. In fact, "greasing the groove," the regimen from Pavel's book, is something that Zak has always done, either instinctually or as a matter of necessity.

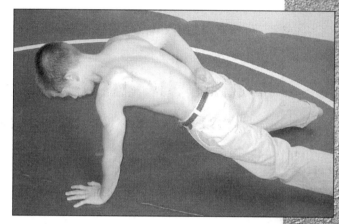

Zak Maxwell, a Naked Warrior. Photo courtesy *maxercise.com*

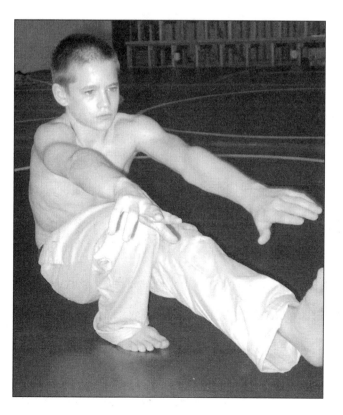

My family lives in a split-level house with a very open floor plan. My wife chose it so that we could keep an eye on the kids from just about anywhere in the house, but what the design of the house is really good for is climbing. While the rest of us use the stairs to get from the living room to the kitchen/dining area, Zak's method has always been to do a wall pull-up on the 6 foot living room half-wall, jump his grip 2 more feet up to the railing and pull himself up again over the railing and into the dining area.

In essence, he is doing two very difficult pull-ups because of the friction of his body dragging on the wall and the lack of gripping purchase on the wall and railing. Multiply this process by the amount of times that a normal kid goes to the refrigerator and you'll see that Zak has been unconsciously employing the GTG technique.

To go to the third floor bathroom, he climbs an 18' rope (yes, the neighbors do think we're a little...different) without his legs to the balcony from the dining room foyer. It takes him between 14 to 15 mini pulls to get to the top.

Consequently, although he rarely performed actual pull-ups on a bar, as an exercise, he came off like a superhero with those 16 pull-ups. The next highest score was 6, which is a reflection of the sad general fitness levels of our school kids, but don't get me started on that one.

My point is that while Zak was periodically performing pistols or one armed-pushups or scaling the wall en route to the refrigerator as a break from the arduous pursuit of Playstation, he was greasing the groove, although neither one of us realized it, which meant that the rest of my clients couldn't enjoy the benefits.

When Pavel identified this technique, it made sense that Zak would be able to execute up to 21 perfect, butt-touch-the-floor pistols, when challenged. Or that in that same 7th grade fitness test, he performed 56 push-ups in 60 seconds, truly the stuff of legend in that school. It also makes sense that although specific abdominal work is rarely included in his workouts, he has a perfect 6-pack. Being lean as a whippet helps, but it is his use of proper tension and breathing techniques during his exercise that makes his abs so pronounced."

Can I add more exercises to the Naked Warrior program?

It's best not to GTG with more than two unrelated exercises, but you may add other exercises that don't overlap much with the pistol and the one-arm pushup. For instance, deadlifts or pullups are good and bench presses are not. Handstand pushups are marginal; they "smoke" many of the muscles heavily involved in the one-arm pushup but in a very different plane. You might try them and see what happens.

To keep it simple, do your other strength exercises, with bodyweight or with iron, two to three times a week for 5x5. Just realize that the more you add to your daily training, the more likely you are to overtrain.

Will my development be unbalanced from doing only two exercises?

Not likely if you follow the instructions. Properly performed, the pistol and the one-arm pushup will challenge most of your major muscle groups. Even your lats will get a workout, if you apply the corkscrew maneuver. Your abs will work hard, too, pressurizing your abdomen and stabilizing you during one-arm pushups.

The areas that will be lacking are the calves, the lower back, the traps, and the forearms. All of these areas (minus the calves) can be addressed with barbell deadlifts or kettlebell snatches. For the calves, jumping rope will do the trick.

Is there a way to work the lats with a pulling exercise when no weights or pullup bars are accessible?

Yes. Let me pass along two excellent anywhere, anytime drills that I learned from two world champion martial artists.

Door Pullups

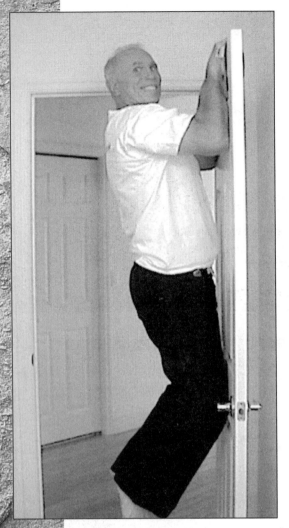

Kickboxing legend Bill "Superfoot" Wallace makes use of his door for a pullup. *Photo courtesy superfoot.com*

The "door pullup" is an invention of professional kickboxing legend Bill Wallace, MS. All you need is a door that's sturdy enough to hold your weight and a ceiling that's tall enough to clear your head. If you were dumb enough to stay at a cheap motel and ripped off the door and crashed, it is your problem, not "Superfoot's".

Open the door and hang onto it, your hands shoulder width apart and your knees bent to clear the floor. You may want to throw a towel over the door. Cramp your glutes to bring your hips closer to the door and pull yourself up.

You will find that your lats get a powerful overload because your elbows are pressed into the door and your elbow flexors have minimal leverage. The friction between your knees and the door will make your lats work even harder. The negative will be easy, but you cannot have it all. You can also do this drill on a wall or a fence.

Door Rows

Rows are among the most important exercise for a BJJ player, says senior world champion Steve Maxwell, MS, RKC Sr., owner of maxercise.com. That's why he improvised this cool towel row in his hotel room.

Open a door and loop a bath towel around the knob. Drape it over the knob on both sides of the door, then pull on both ends from below so the towel gets jammed in place. If your door has those small balls pretending to be a doorknob, you will have a problem with the towel slipping. Your luggage shoulder strap will save the day, use it instead of a towel.

The odds are, the bathroom door will not be up to the task and you will have to use your room's front door. Enjoy the publicity. Grab the ends of the towel and face the edge of the door standing a foot or so away from it. Squat down slightly, carefully hang back on the towel, your arms straight. Be ready to recover if the towel slips. Wear shoes so your feet would not slip. Row!

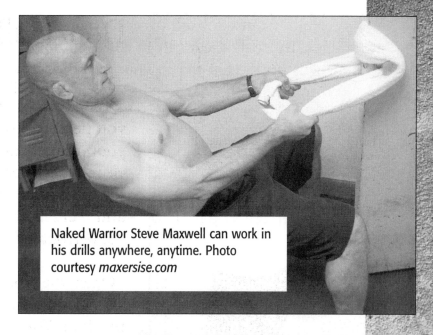

Naked Warrior Steve Maxwell can work in his drills anywhere, anytime. Photo courtesy *maxersise.com*

The drill is highly versatile. Here is how to customize it. The resistance may be easily adjusted by redistributing your weight between your feet and your hands. Try squatting down, standing up, moving your feet closer or further from the door; play with it. Super studs may try the one arm version of the doorknob towel row. Holding both ends of the towel in one hand will also give you a grip workout to write home about. A halfway there option is to row with both arms while keeping more weight on one of them. The door will squeak from uneven pressure. Deal with it.

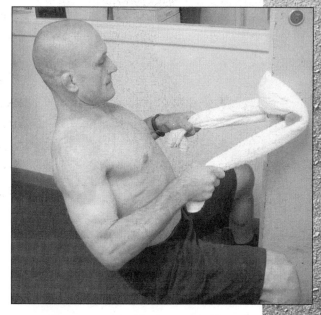

Although the row could be adapted to stress your lats and other pulling muscles at different angles by leaning way forward (feels like a pullup) or way back (feels like an upright row), it is not recommended. Unless you are in a natural semi-squat and nearly upright, you would put yourself into a precarious position in case the towel or your feet slip. So stick with the basic row.

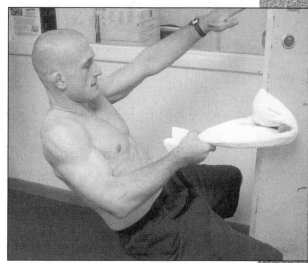

189

Pull "from the back of your armpits" to assure that you are working your lats. Pause momentarily in the beginning and in the end of the movement and focus on the tension in your "wings". Try to maintain that tension steadily throughout the rep, all the way until your elbows are locked. No silly half-reps, Comrade; lock those elbows!

The position of your elbows also makes a difference. Keeping them very high targets the rear delts. It is best to drop your elbows slightly for your lats. Breathe in as you row, breathe out as you straighten out your arms. It is most natural with this exercise.

Grab the towel with an over grip, as the row progresses, supinate your hands so the palms are facing up by the time they are by your sides. Like a karate punch. The sets and reps are up to you; as you would expect, I would limit the reps to 5 and do more sets. It's a great idea to alternate or superset the towel rows with some sort of a pushup.

How should I apply the Naked Warrior techniques to my sport-specific conditioning?

The answer to this question lies outside the scope of this book. Let your coach or at least your common sense be your guide.

Where can I learn more about bodyweight-only strength training?

My publisher's website, dragondoor.com, boasts many excellent articles on a wide range of topics: bodyweight strength training, kettlebell training, strength training and powerlifting, conditioning, tactical and martial arts, and martial arts and close-quarter combat skills. It's free to access any of the articles; all you have to do is click on "Articles" and then subscribe to my *Power by Pavel* newsletter (which is also free). My newsletter has more free training information than promotion.

Following is an example of training advice from my newsletter:

Com. John Du Cane, RKC, author of *The Five Animal Frolics,* has shown me the "wall squat", a variation of the bodyweight squat popular with Chinese Chi Kung practitioners. In addition to its health benefits, the drill will teach you how to lock your lower back in as tight as an expert powerlifter. And it will loosen it up big time in the process.

Stand a couple of inches away from a wall facing it, your arms hanging free as if you are about to deadlift. Keep your feet parallel and close to each other. Squat as low as you can, try to work into a full squat. You must stand as close to the wall as possible; your forehead should be almost brushing it. Something cool will happen in your lower back when your hips are almost parallel to the deck; you cannot miss it.

Comrades who are very strong: challenge yourselves with wall pistols. Stand by a corner so the knee of your working leg and your head are blocked by the wall yet your airborne leg is free to go straight around the corner.

Low reps and no failure? This training is too easy!

Don't complain that high-tension training doesn't build character. It wasn't meant to. Its laser-sharp focus is strength.

But if you're looking for lesson in character building, when you are done with your strength practice, go test your mettle with a few high-rep sets of kettlebell snatches. "This is the hardest thing I have done in my life," said one Recon Marine after making his acquaintance with the Russian kettlebell. Try it, if you think you are so tough. You will wish you were dead.

Will I forget all the strength techniques in some sort of emergency?

"Under stress, we revert to our training". This is an axiom in the military and law enforcement communities. If you have been practicing the right moves a lot, when your adrenalin kicks in, you will do the right thing on autopilot. Or the wrong thing, depending on what you have been practicing.

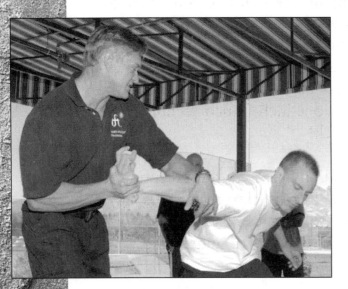

"Under stress we revert to training," says close quarter combat expert Tim Larkin, RKC. Photo courtesy tftgroup.com

Tim Larkin, RKC, formerly Special Warfare Intelligence Officer for the Naval admiral in charge of all SEAL Teams and currently a hand-to-hand combat instructor to spec ops units and civilians (see tftgroup.com for details of Tim's outstanding courses), likes to tell a story about a cleanliness-obsessed police range master who hated having loose brass lying around his spotless firing range. He insisted that the officers put the spent cartridges from their revolvers into their pockets while they were practicing. Then two cops got killed in a shootout. And guess what? They were found with their hands clutching empty shells in their pockets. Had they dropped the brass, they could have stayed alive.

By the same token, proper combat reloads, if practiced, also "just happen" in life-and-death situations. If you perform any action consciously enough times, it will become automatic.

Likewise, high-tension techniques can be hard wired into your spinal cord through diligent practice. Practice enough, and your abs will automatically tighten up when they are needed. This principle, along with all the others in *The Naked Warrior*, has worked for generations of martial artists.

Isn't dedicating most of the book to technique too much?

Strength is technique. When someone told Bulgarian weightlifting coach Angel Spassov that his training was "not normal," he quipped, "Who wants to be normal? We choose to be extraordinary."

The same goes for the Naked Warrior program. Typical books on strength training shrug off the issue of strength technique by telling you to "emphasize the negative, don't jerk, don't arch, inhale on the way down and exhale on the way up." While these pointers might be easy to remember, following them will bring you only typical—read "marginal at best"—results. Using the martial arts analogy, it's like explaining the one-inch punch technique by saying, "Punch from an inch away." Good luck!

Maximum power generation is a science and an art. With the exception of a few talented superathletes, who "just do it," the top performers have reached the top by relentlessly honing their technique. Bench press world champion George Halbert said that it took him 13 years to understand what the triceps really do in the bench press!

If you aren't willing to apply this level of attention and patience to your strength training, then learn to be content with being weak. Pick out one of the many sissified programs floating around or sign up for a "muscle-conditioning" class at your local health spa and get "fit"—whatever that means. Tell them sissies hello.

A Parting Shot...There Are No Excuses!

Suren Bogdasarov, a Soviet army officer and coach of legendary weightlifting champion Yuri Vlasov, was promoting strength training in the armed forces in the late 1970s/early 1980s. At one unit, he heard someone complain that they did not have the proper equipment.

"I took two chairs," reminisces the great coach, "and set them down a shoulder width apart with the backs facing in. Then I started doing dips on the chairs' backs...After 8–10 dips, I did abdominal work. I lifted straight legs to my shoulder level, then lowered them while maintaining the L-seat. Then I climbed up on a chair with one foot and started doing one-legged squats. I stepped off the chair and did jumping good mornings, it is a forward bend followed by a back bend and finished with a jump. After all this I showed them a few more bodyweight exercises."

Bogdasarov, a man addicted to iron, will never quit lifting barbells and kettlebells. But he is even more hooked on strength and will not settle for doing nothing when his beloved heavy metal isn't around. As this Naked Warrior said when he finished his presentation, "One must use any means in his disposal and not wait for manna from heaven."

Power to you! Anywhere. Anytime. With or without hardware.

Power to you, Naked Warrior!

Pavel

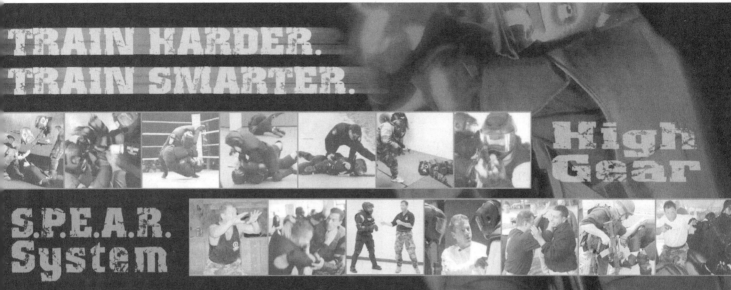
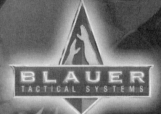

ABOUT PAVEL

Pavel Tsatsouline, Master of
Sports, is a former Soviet Special
Forces instructor and a
nationally ranked athlete in the
Russian military applied sport of
kettlebell lifting.

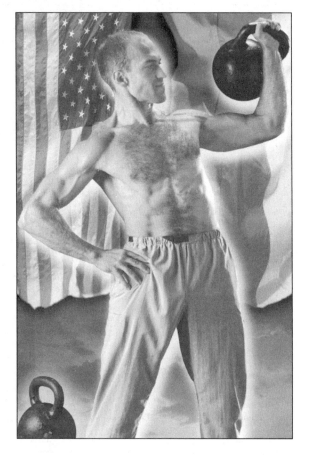

Today Pavel is a subject matter
expert to the US Marine Corps,
the US Secret Service, and federal
nuclear security teams. He
makes his "low tech/high
concepts" strength and flexibility
techniques available to civilians
through his bestselling books and
videos from Dragon Door
Publications.

Rolling Stone's 'Hot Trainer',
Pavel has been interviewed by
CNN Headline News, the Fox News Channel, and the Associated Press and
featured in media ranging from *Wall Street Journal* to *Pravda*.

How to stay informed of the latest advances in strength and conditioning
VISIT WWW.HARD-STYLE.COM

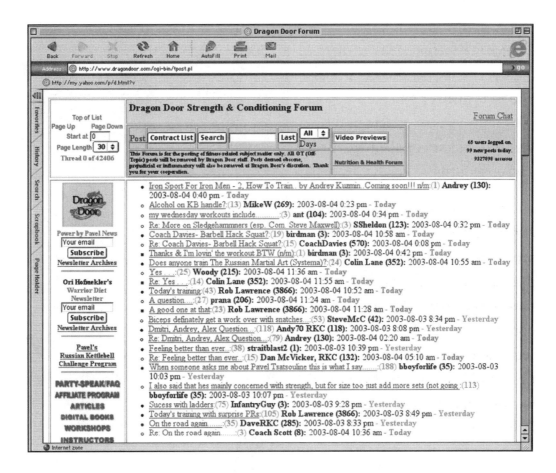

Visit **www.hard-style.com** and sign up for Pavel Tsatsouline's free monthly e-newsletter, giving you late-breaking news and tips on how to stay ahead of the fitness pack.

Visit **www.dragondoor.com/cgi-bin/tpost.pl** and participate in Dragon Door's stimulating and informative **Strength and Conditioning** Forum. Post your fitness questions or comments and get quick feedback from Pavel Tsatsouline and other leading fitness experts.

Visit **www.dragondoor.com** and browse the **Articles** section and other pages for groundbreaking theories and products for improving your health and well being.

The Graduate Course In Instant Strength Gain

"I went from 5 to 10 pullups in one week."

"Last night I did 15 one-arm pushups with each arm. Two months ago I couldn't do one complete rep."

"I could do one wobbly one-legged squat... [Two weeks later] I did 5 clean, butt-to-ground pistols."

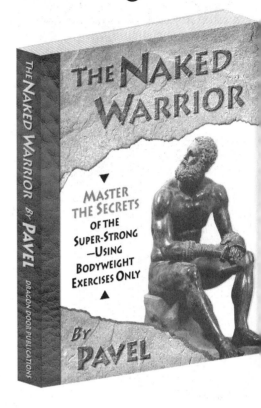

Have you noticed—the greater a man's skill, the more he achieves with less? And the skill of strength is no exception. From the ancient days of Greek wrestling, to the jealously guarded secrets of Chinese Kung Fu masters, to the hard men of modern spec ops, warriors and allied strongmen have developed an amazing array of skills for generating inhuman strength.

But these skills have been scattered far and wide, held closely secret, or communicated in a piecemeal fashion that has left most of us frustrated and far from reaching our true strength potential.

Now, for the first time, Russian strength expert and former *Spetsnaz* instructor Pavel has gathered many of these devastating techniques into one highly teachable skill set. In *The Naked Warrior* Pavel reveals exactly what it takes to be super-strong in minimum time—when your body is your only tool.

- Gain more brute strength in days than you did in years of bodybuilding or calisthenics
- Discover the martial secrets of instant power generation—for rapid surges in applied strength
- Discover how to get a world-class powerlifter's quality workout—using your body only
- Get a harder, firmer, functionally-fitter body—and be as resilient as hell whatever you face

- Master the one-arm/one-leg pushup for crushing upper body force
- Forge super-piston, never-quit legs with the Spetsnaz favorite "Pistol"
- Discover the magic of "GTG"—guaranteed the world's most effective strength routine
- Be tow-truck strong—yet possess the rugged looks of a stripped-down racer
- No gym, no weights, no problem—get a dynamite strength workout at a moment's notice—wherever you are

The Naked Warrior
Master the Secrets of the Super-Strong—Using Bodyweight Exercises Only
By Pavel
#B28 $39.95
Paperback 218 pages 8.5" x 11"
Over 190 black & white photos plus several illustrations

"Pavel's Naked Warrior DVD is worth its weight in gold!"

"The Naked Warrior DVD is worth its weight in gold! I just completed several honest one arm pushups after viewing the NW DVD. Despite reading the book and practicing, I just couldn't make it happen. I watched the DVD and finally understood that I was letting my shoulder drift. Tightened up and several honest square-to-the-floor one arm pushups were mine!!"—siameeser, dragondoor.com forum, 5/13/04

"NW DVD is fantastic ! I had the book & have been working toward full range pistols and OAPUs for a while. A HUGE help to see Pavel doing the movements. Results: Before watching DVD - I could do 2 OAPUs on a good day with so-so form. First workout after watching DVD: 1 set of 3 and 2 sets of 2 with good form. For pistols (at about a foot off the floor). Before I watched the DVD - 2 reps with shaky form. First workout after watching DVD - 2 sets of 5 and one set of 4 solid. Very impressed with DVD - thanks Com. Pavel."— dkaler, dragondoor.com forum, 5/17/04

The Naked Warrior
Master the Secrets of the Super-Strong—Using Bodyweight Exercises Only with Pavel
DVD #DV015 $34.95
Video #V114 $34.95
Running time 37 minutes

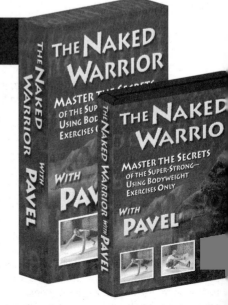

"Discover How to Reinforce Your Body—and Snap Back from the Toughest Challenge with Deceptive Ease and Strength"

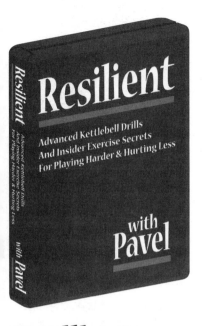

Life has a habit of body-slamming us when we least expect it. And the more active we are, the more likely we're gonna be wrenched, tossed, torn, torqued, twisted, scrunched, hammered and generally whacked around. Hit your forties—let alone fifties—and you can be reduced to a tangled mess of injuries and performance-crimping tensions.

You get sidelined! You can't do what you want to do anymore. People don't want you on their team anymore. You can't compete anymore. You're... let's face it...washed up, as a card-carrying member of the active elite. Sometimes all it takes is one sudden injury to that one weak spot you neglected to strengthen and defend....and you're history.

As a former *Spetsnaz* physical training instructor

and as a current subject-matter expert to elite members of the U.S. military, **Pavel** knows what it takes—personally and professionally—to remove flaws and weaknesses from your body armor—so you can bounce back, time and time again, from the toughest challenge.

So, in this specialized program, Pavel's put together 19 of his favorite drills for restoring and reinforcing your body's "rebound strength." Pavel's concentrated on the weak links—the knees, the elbows, the shoulders, the spine, the neck—and shows you how to change a liability-waiting-to-happen into a strength-weapon-of-choice.

Discover what it really means to be RESILIENT. Add years of wiry, tensile, pliant strength back into your life—and hurt a whole lot less while you're doing it.

Resilient
Advanced Kettlebell Drills and Insider Secrets for Playing Harder & Hurting Less
with Pavel
#DV017 DVD $59.95
Running time: 36 minutes

Pavel's Resilient program:

- **Develops** a more flexible, yet stronger neck
- **Restores** crucial elbow strength and mobility
- **Develops** spectacular shoulder girdle and upper back flexibility
- **Boosts** performance for girevoy sport, weightlifting, powerlifting, strongman events, gymnastics, yoga
- **Loosens** up your spine while teaching you powerful body mechanics
- **Rewards** you with the ultimate in squatting flexibility—a must for military and law enforcement

- **Helps** you move like liquid metal
- **Conditions** your knees in a little-known plane that can spell the difference between true resilience and dangerous weakness
- **Helps** release your tight hip flexors—which act like parking brakes to cripple your kicking, punching, running and lifting
- **Develops** a stronger, more sinuous back
- **Stretches** your spine—for extra "activity-mileage"
- **Injury-proofs** your back with a little-knownl drill from Russian contact sports

Customer reviews from Dragon Door's website

"Worth every penny! This DVD is probably the best I have ever viewed. The moves for the shoulders are excellent, the RKC arm bar, the triceps extension, and the one that really surprised me the most was the hack shoulder stretch was the best and made an immediate impact on my shoulders. Keep up the good work."
—Donnie, West Hamlin, WV

"Concise and truly beneficial. Pavel breaks these drills down wonderfully: first demonstrating, then focusing on finer points and offering visualizations for safety, power, and keeping form. As a member of a special reaction team, our training requires performance in any condition. Pavel's products and drills like these

help keep me mobile and ready. A great DVD!"
—Michael Ottaway, FE Warren AFB, WY

"Ever get beat up? I had one of those months. Between wrestling, brazilian jiu-jitsu, training for the Washington State Kettlebell Championships and the June 2004 RKC, I was run down and hurting. Just lots of hard training, plus getting bounced off the mat 100 times a day in my takedown class I felt like everything hurt. So I took a month, and all I did was Resilient exercises with my 26 lb kettlebell, Super Joints, and a little juggling with my 26 lb kettlebell. All my joints feel SOOOOO GOOD. Coming back I feel stronger and more solid everywhere. Now I'm still doing the

Resilient exercises as preventive medicine. The neck stuff is REALLY good for my Brazilian Jiu Jitsu."
—Joshua Hillis RKC, NASM-CPT - Denver, CO

"If as a male, you thought 8kg or 12kg KB were for women only? I strongly suggest you think again. With this product, Pavel shows, yet again the information you need to "re-install & repair" your joints. Nothing's a patch on Pavel. In fact, I wonder if I went to the Australian Government & asked for my HECS fees back, if they'd agree. I spent four years at Uni with a double major in Physical Education, yet this information was not provided!"
—Pete Rogers, Hobart, Tasmania

"Discover How to Reinforce Your Body— and Snap Back from the Toughest Challenge with Deceptive Ease and Strength"

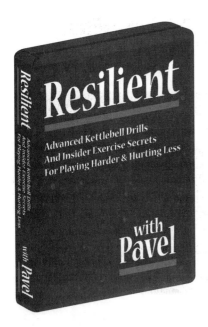

Life has a habit of body-slamming us when we least expect it. And the more active we are, the more likely we're gonna be wrenched, tossed, torn, torqued, twisted, scrunched, hammered and generally whacked around. Hit your forties—let alone fifties—and you can be reduced to a tangled mess of injuries and performance-crimping tensions.

You get sidelined! You can't do what you want to do anymore. People don't want you on their team anymore. You can't compete anymore. You're... let's face it...washed up, as a card-carrying member of the active elite. Sometimes all it takes is one sudden injury to that one weak spot you neglected to strengthen and defend....and you're history.

As a former *Spetsnaz* physical training instructor and as a current subject-matter expert to elite members of the U.S. military, **Pavel** knows what it takes—personally and professionally—to remove flaws and weaknesses from your body armor—so you can bounce back, time and time again, from the toughest challenge.

So, in this specialized program, Pavel's put together 19 of his favorite drills for restoring and reinforcing your body's "rebound strength." Pavel's concentrated on the weak links—the knees, the elbows, the shoulders, the spine, the neck—and shows you how to change a liability-waiting-to-happen into a strength-weapon-of-choice.

Discover what it really means to be RESILIENT. Add years of wiry, tensile, pliant strength back into your life—and hurt a whole lot less while you're doing it.

Resilient
Advanced Kettlebell Drills and Insider Secrets for Playing Harder & Hurting Less
with Pavel
#DV017 DVD $59.95
Running time: 36 minutes

Pavel's Resilient program:

- **Develops a more flexible, yet stronger neck**
- **Restores crucial elbow strength and mobility**
- **Develops spectacular shoulder girdle and upper back flexibility**
- **Boosts performance for girevoy sport, weightlifting, powerlifting, strongman events, gymnastics, yoga**
- **Loosens up your spine while teaching you powerful body mechanics**
- **Rewards you with the ultimate in squatting flexibility—a must for military and law enforcement**

- **Helps you move like liquid metal**
- **Conditions your knees in a little-known plane that can spell the difference between true resilience and dangerous weakness**
- **Helps release your tight hip flexors—which act like parking brakes to cripple your kicking, punching, running and lifting**
- **Develops a stronger, more sinuous back**
- **Stretches your spine—for extra "activity-mileage"**
- **Injury-proofs your back with a little-knownl drill from Russian contact sports**

Customer reviews from Dragon Door's website

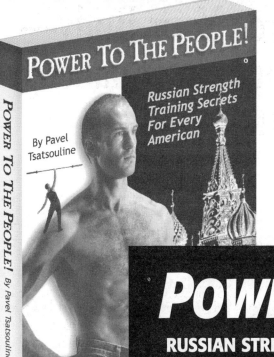

"*Power to the People!* is absolute dynamite. If there was only one book I could recommend to help you reach your ultimate physical potential, this would be it."

—Jim Wright, Ph.D., Science Editor, Flex Magazine, Weider Group

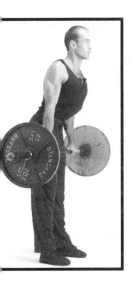

How would you like to own a world class body—<u>whatever your present condition</u>— by doing only two exercises, for twenty minutes a day?"   A body so lean, ripped and powerful looking, you won't believe your own reflection when you catch yourself in the mirror.

And what if you could do it without a single supplement, without having to waste your time at a gym and with only a 150 bucks of simple equipment?

And how about not only being stronger than you've ever been in your life, but having higher energy and better performance in whatever you do?

How would you like to have an instant download of the world's <u>absolutely most effective strength secrets?</u> To possess exactly the same knowledge that created world-champion athletes—and the strongest bodies of their generation?"

Pavel Tsatsouline's *Power to the People!– Russian Strength Training Secrets for Every American* delivers all of this and more.

As **Senior Science Editor for Joe Weider's *Flex*** magazine, Jim Wright is recognized as one of the world's premier authorities on strength training. Here's more of what he had to say:

"*Whether you're young or old, a beginner or an elite athlete, training in your room or in the most high tech facility, if there was only one book I could recommend to help you reach your ultimate physical potential, this would be it.*

Simple, concise and truly reader friendly, this amazing book contains it all—everything you need to know—what exercises (only two!), how to do them (unique detailed information you'll find nowhere else), and why.

Follow its advice and, believe it or not, you'll be stronger and more injury-resistant immediately. I guarantee it. I only wish I'd had a book like this when I first began training.

Follow this program for three months and you'll not only be amazed but hooked. It is the ultimate program for "Everyman" AND Woman! I thought I knew a lot with a Ph.D. and 40 years of training experience...but I learned a lot and it's improved my training significantly."

And how about this from **World Masters Powerlifting champion and Parrillo Performance Press editor, Marty Gallagher:**

"*Pavel Tsatsouline has burst onto the American health and fitness scene like a Russian cyclone. He razes the sacred temples of fitness complacency and smugness with his revolutionary concepts and ideas. If you want a new and innovative approach to the age old dilemma of physical transformation, you've struck the mother-lode.*"

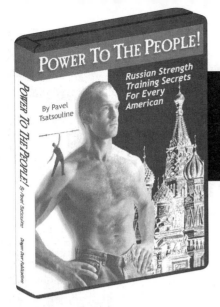

Now, It's Yours for the Taking:

IRRESISTIBLE STRENGTH and a BODY-TO-DIE-FOR

Turn on Pavel's *Power to the People!* video

and watch in amazement as you rapidly increase your strength by 20, 30, even 50 percent—often in one session!

Power to the People!

Russian Strength Secrets for Every American **Video**

With Pavel Tsatsouline

Running Time 47 Min

DVD **#DV004 $29.95**

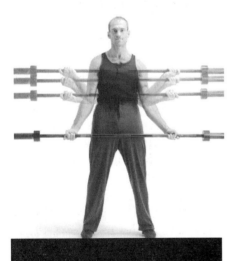

Whatever your current workout program, just download Pavel's strength techniques for an immediate improvement in your results.

You may, or may not, want to startle your friends, excite your lovers, scare your enemies and paralyze your neighbors with envy, but believe me, it's gonna happen when you easily absorb Pavel's breakthrough strength secrets.

Of course, what's most important is how you're gonna feel about yourself. Get real! Toss out your lame rationalizations and pathetic excuses. Stop behaving like a spoilt brat about your infantile levels of strength. Stop hating yourself for banging your head against phony training plateaus. Now you can smash through the glass ceiling of your ignorance and burst into the higher reaches of maximum performance.

Let's face it—it's a delicious feeling to be as strong as a panther—confident, sure-of-yourself, genuinely attractive, a <u>SPECIMEN, THE GENUINE ARTICLE</u>, stalking the streets with evident power and natural grace.

I don't care who you are or what you are, I promise you: grab Pavel's Power to the People! video <u>IMMEDIATELY</u>, plug yourself in—and <u>I MEAN, PLUG YOURSELF IN</u>—do what it says, and you won't believe the new you.

- Achieve super-strength without training to muscle failure or exhaustion
- Know the secret of hacking into your 'muscle software' to magnify power and muscle

- Get super strong without putting on an ounce of weight
- Discover what it really takes to develop spectacular muscle tone
- Discover how to mold your whole body into an off-planet rock with only two exercises
- Now you can design a world class body in your basement—with $150 worth of basic weights and in twenty minutes a day
- Discover futuristic techniques to squeeze more horsepower out of your body-engine
- Discover how to maximize muscular tension and get traffic-stopping muscular definition
- Learn why it's safer to use free weights than machines
- How to achieve massive muscles and awesome strength—if that's what you want
- How to master the magic of effective exercise variation
- Know how to gain beyond your wildest dreams—with less chance of injury
- Discover a high intensity, immediate gratification technique for massive strength gains
- Discover the eight most effective breathing habits for lifting weights
- Learn the secret that separates elite athletes from 'also-rans'

If you are looking for a
SUPREME EDGE
in your chosen sport —seek no more!

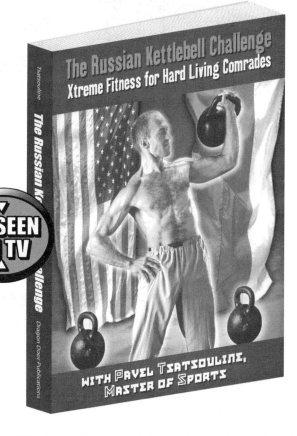

AS SEEN ON TV

The Russian Kettlebell Challenge–Xtreme Fitness for Hard Living Comrades

Book By Pavel Tsatsouline

#B15 *$34.95* Paperback 170 pages

With Pavel Tsatsouline

Running Time: 32 minutes

Video *#V103* *$39.95*

DVD *#DV001* *$39.95*

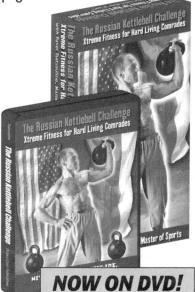

NOW ON DVD!

Both the Soviet Special Forces and numerous world-champion Soviet Olympic athletes used the ancient Russian Kettlebells as their secret weapon for xtreme fitness. Thanks to the kettlebell's astonishing ability to turbocharge physical performance, these Soviet supermen creamed their opponents time-and-time again, with inhuman displays of raw power and explosive strength.

Now, former Spetznaz trainer, international fitness author and nationally-ranked kettlebell lifter, Pavel Tsatsouline, delivers this secret Soviet weapon into your own hands. You NEVER have to be second best again! Here is the first-ever complete kettlebell training program—for Western shock-attack athletes who refuse to be denied—and who'd rather be dead than number two.

- *Get* really, really nasty—with a commando's wiry strength, the explosive agility of a tiger and the stamina of a world-class ironman
- *Own* the single best conditioning tool for killer sports like kickboxing, wrestling, and football
- *Watch* in amazement as high-rep kettlebells let you hack the fat off your meat—without the dishonor of aerobics and dieting
- *Kick* your fighting system into warp speed—with high-rep snatches and clean-and-jerks
- *Develop* steel tendons and ligaments—with a whiplash power to match
- *Effortlessly absorb* ballistic shocks—and laugh as you shrug off the hardest hits your opponent can muster
- *Go ape* on your enemies—with gorilla shoulders and tree-swinging traps

"Pavel started a veritable revolution, no less, when this book came out…" —Randall Strossen, Ph. D., *Iron Mind Enterprises*, ironmind.com

"In *The Russian Kettlebell Challenge*, Pavel Tsatsouline presents a masterful treatise on a superb old-time training tool and the unique exercises that yielded true strength and endurance to the rugged pioneers of the iron game. Proven infinitely more efficient than any fancy modern exercise apparatus, the kettlebell via Pavel's recommendations is adaptable to numerous high and low rep schemes to offer any strength athlete, bodybuilder, martial artist, or sports competitor a superior training regimen. As a former International General Secretary of the International All-Round Weightlifting Association, I not only urge all athletes to study Mr. Tsatsouline's book and try these wonderful all-round kettlebell movements, but plan to recommend that many kettlebell lifts again become part of our competitions!" —John McKean, current IAWA world and national middleweight champion

"Everybody with an interest in the serious matter of body regulation over a lifetime should commit themselves to Pavel's genre of knowledge and his distinct techniques of writing. Any one of the dozens of suggestions you hit upon will pay for the *Russian Kettlebell Challenge* hundreds of times." —Len Schwartz, author of *Heavyhands: the Ultimate Exercise System* and *The Heavyhands*

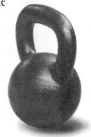

RUSSIAN KETTLEBELLS

The World's #1 Handheld Gym For Extreme Fitness

Use Kettlebells to:

- **Accelerate your all-purpose strength**—so you can readily handle the toughest demands
- **Hack away your fat**—without the dishonor of dieting and aerobics
- **Boost your physical resilience**—to repel the hardest hits
- **Build your staying power**—to endure and conquer, whatever the distance
- **Create a potent mix of strength-with-flexibility**—to always reach your target
- **Forge a fighter's physique**—so form matches function
- **Be independent**—world's #1 portable gym makes you as strong as you want to be, anywhere, anytime

Kettlebells Fly Air Force One!

"There's a competitive reason behind the appearance of kettlebells at the back doors and tent flaps of military personnel. When Russian and US Special Forces started competing against each other after the Soviet Union broke up, the Americans made a disturbing discovery. "We'd be totally exhausted and the Russians wouldn't even be catching their breath," says... [a] Secret Service agent... "It turned out they were all working with kettlebells."

Now, half the Secret Service is snatching kettlebells and a set sometimes travels with the President's detail on Air Force One. *Christian Science Monitor*

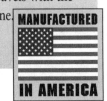

Pavel's Kettlebell FAQ

What is a 'kettlebell'?

A 'kettlebell' or girya (Russ.) is a traditional Russian cast iron wei that looks like a cannonball with a handle. The ultimate tool extreme all-round fitness.

The kettlebell goes way back – it first appeared in a Russ dictionary in 1704 (Cherkikh, 1994). So popular were kettlebell Tsarist Russia that any strongman or weightlifter was referred to a girevik, or 'a kettlebell man'.

"Not a single sport develops our muscular strength and bodies as w as kettlebell athletics," reported Russian magazine Hercules in 191

"Kettlebells—Hot Weight of the Year"—Rolling Stone

Why train with kettlebells?

Because they deliver extreme all-round fitness. And no single o tool does it better. Here is a short list of hardware the Russian kettle replaces: barbells, dumbbells, belts for weighted pullups and dips, t bars, lever bars, medicine balls, grip devices, and cardio equipment

Vinogradov & Lukyanov (1986) found a very high correla between the results posted in a kettlebell lifting competition and a g range of dissimilar tests: strength, measured with the three power and grip strength; strength endurance, measured with pullups parallel bar dips; general endurance, determined by a 1000 meter work capacity and balance, measured with special tests.

Voropayev (1983) tested two groups of subjects in pullups, a stan broad jump, a 100m sprint, and a 1k run. He put the control grou a program that emphasized the above tests; the experimental gr lifted kettlebells. In spite of the lack of practice on the tested exerc the kettlebell group scored better in every one of them! This is wha call "the what the hell effect".

Kettlebells melt fat without the dishonor of dieting or aerobics. If are overweight, you will lean out. If you are skinny, you will get up. According to Voropayev (1997) who studied top Russian girev 21.2% increased their bodyweight since taking up kettlebelling 21.2% (the exact same percentage, not a typo), mostly heavyweig decreased it. The Russian kettlebell is a powerful tool for fixing y body comp, whichever way it needs fixing.

Kettlebells forge doers' physiques along the lines of antique sta broad shoulders with just a hint of pecs, back muscles standing o bold relief, wiry arms, rugged forearms, a cut-up midsection, and str legs without a hint of squatter's chafing.

Liberating and aggressive as medieval swordplay, kettlebell trai is highly addictive. What other piece of exercise equipment can b that its owners name it? Paint it? Get tattoos of it? Our Rus kettlebell is the Harley-Davidson of strength hardware.

"Kettlebells—A Workout with Balls"—Men's Journal

Who trains with kettlebells?

Hard comrades of all persuasions.

Soviet weightlifting legends such as Vlasov, Zhabotinskiy, and Alexeyev started their Olympic careers with old-fashioned kettlebells. Yuri Vlasov once interrupted an interview he was giving to a Western journalist and proceeded to press a pair of kettlebells. "A wonderful exercise," commented the world champion. "...It is hard to find an exercise better suited for developing strength and flexibility simultaneously."

The Russian Special Forces personnel owe much of their wiry strength, explosive agility, and never-quitting stamina to kettlebells. *Soldier, Be Strong!*, the official Soviet armed forces strength training manual pronounced kettlebell drills to be "one of the most effective means of strength development" representing "a new era in the development of human strength-potential".

The elite of the US military and law enforcement instantly recognized the power of the Russian kettlebell, ruggedly simple and deadly effective as an AK-47. You can find Pavel's certified RKC instructors among Force Recon Marines, Department of Energy nuclear security teams, the FBI's Hostage Rescue Team, the Secret Service Counter Assault Team, etc.

Once the Russian kettlebell became a hit among those whose life depends on their strength and conditioning, it took off among hard people from all walks of life: martial artists, athletes, regular hard comrades.

"I can't think of a more practical way of special operations training... I was extremely skeptical about kettlebell training and now wish that I had known about it fifteen years ago..."

—*Name withheld, Special Agent, U.S. Secret Service Counter Assault Team*

Am I kettlebell material?

Kettlebell training is extreme but not elitist. At the 1995 Russian Championship the youngest contestant was 16, the oldest 53! And we are talking elite competition here; the range is even wider if you are training for yourself rather than for the gold. Dr. Krayevskiy, the father of the kettlebell sport, took up training at the age of forty-one and twenty years later he was said to look fresher and healthier than at forty.

Only 8.8% of top Russian gireviks, members of the Russian National Team and regional teams, reported injuries in training or competition (Voropayev, 1997). A remarkably low number, especially if you consider that these are elite athletes who push their bodies over the edge. Many hard men with high mileage have overcome debilitating injuries with kettlebell training (get your doctor's approval). Acrobat Valentin Dikul fell and broke his back at seventeen. Today, in his mid-sixties, he juggles 180-pound balls and breaks powerlifting records!

"... kettlebells are a unique conditioning tool and a powerful one as well that you should add to your arsenal of strength... my experience with them has been part of what's led me to a modification in my thoughts on strength and bodyweight exercises... I'm having a blast training with them and I think you will as well."

—Bud Jeffries, the author of *How to Squat 900lbs. without Drugs, Powersuits, or Kneewraps*

How do I learn to use the kettlebell?

From Pavel's books and videos: *The Russian Kettlebell Challenge* or *From Russia with Tough Love* for comrades ladies. From an RKC certified instructor; find one in your area on RussianKettlebell.com. Kettlebell technique can be learned in one or two sessions and you can start intense training during the second or even first week (Dvorkin, 2001).

"...I felt rejuvenated and ready to conquer the world. I was sold on the kettlebells, as the exercises were fun and challenging, and demanded coordination, explosion, balance, and power... I am now on my way to being a better, fitter, and more explosive grappler, and doing things I haven't done in years!"

—Kid Peligro, *Grappling* magazine

What is the right kettlebell size for me?

Kettlebells come in 'poods'. A pood is an old Russian measure of weight, which equals 16kg, or roughly 35 lbs. An average man should start with a 35-pounder. It does not sound like a lot but believe it; it feels a lot heavier than it should! Most men will eventually progress to a 53-pounder, the standard issue size in the Russian military. Although available in most units, 70-pounders are used only by a few advanced guys and in elite competitions. 88-pounders are for mutants.

An average woman should start with an 18-pounder. A strong woman can go for a 26-pounder. Some women will advance to a 35-pounder. A few hard women will go beyond.

"Kettlebells are like weightlifting times ten."

"Kettlebells are like weightlifting times ten. ...If I could've met Pavel in the early '80s, I might've won two gold medals. I'm serious."

—Dennis Koslowski, D.C., RKC, *Olympic Silver Medalist in Greco-Roman Wrestling*

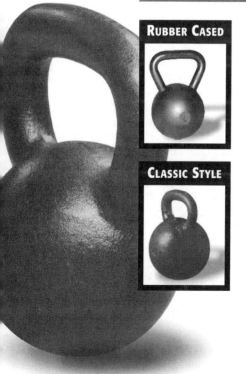

RUBBER CASED

CLASSIC STYLE

STEEL HANDLE & CORE/RUBBER CASING	Price	MAIN USA	AK&HI	CAN
#P10D 4kg (approx. 9lb) −.25 poods	$89.95	S/H $10.00	$52.00	$29.00
#P10E 8kg (approx. 18lb) − .50 poods	$99.95	S/H $14.00	$70.00	$41.00

CLASSIC KETTLEBELLS (SOLID CAST IRON)

	Price	MAIN USA	AK&HI	CAN
#P10G 12kg (approx. 26lb) − .75 poods	$82.95	S/H $20.00	$86.00	$53.00
#P10A 16kg (approx. 35lb) − 1 pood	$89.95	S/H $24.00	$95.00	$65.00
#P10H 20kg (approx. 44lb) − 1.25 poods	$99.95	S/H $28.00	$118.00	$72.00
#P10B 24kg (approx. 53lb) − 1.5 poods	$109.95	S/H $32.00	$137.00	$89.00
#P10J 28kg (approx. 62lb) − 1.75 poods	$129.95	S/H $36.00	$154.00	$102.00
#P10C 32kg (approx. 70lb) − 2 poods	$139.95	S/H $39.00	$173.00	$115.00
#P10F 40kg (approx. 88lb) − 2.5 poods	$179.95	S/H $52.00	$210.00	$139.00

SAVE! ORDER A SET OF CLASSIC KETTLEBELLS & SAVE $17.00

#SP10 Classic Set (one each of 16, 24 & 32kg)	$322.85	S/H $95.00	$405.00	$269.00

ALASKA/HAWAII KETTLEBELL ORDERING
Dragon Door now ships to all 50 states, including Alaska and Hawaii. We ship Kettlebells to Alaska and Hawaii via UPS 2nd Day Air service.

CANADIAN KETTLEBELL ORDERING
Dragon Door now accepts online, phone and mail orders for Kettlebells to Canada, using UPS Standard service. UPS Standard to Canada service is guaranteed, fully tracked ground delivery, available to every address in all of Canada's ten provinces. Delivery time can vary between 3 to 10 days.

IMPORTANT — International shipping quotes & orders do not include customs clearance, duties, taxes or other non-routine customs brokerage charges, which are the responsibility of the customer.

- **KETTLEBELLS ARE SHIPPED VIA UPS GROUND SERVICE, UNLESS OTHERWISE REQUESTED.**
- **KETTLEBELLS RANGING IN SIZE FROM 4KG TO 24KG CAN BE SHIPPED TO P.O. BOXES OR MILITARY ADDDRESSES VIA THE U.S. POSTAL SERVICE, BUT WE REQUIRE PHYSICAL ADDDRESSES FOR UPS DELIVERIES FOR THE 32KG AND 40KG KETTLEBELLS.**
- **NO RUSH ORDERS ON KETTLEBELLS!**

"Download this tape into your eager cells and watch in stunned disbelief as your body reconstitutes itself, almost overnight"

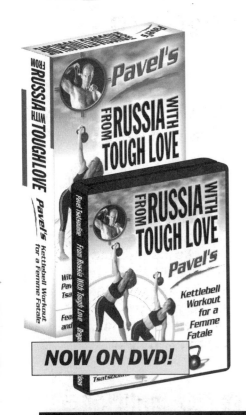

NOW ON DVD!

From Russia with Tough Love

Pavel's Kettlebell Workout
for a Femme Fatale
With Pavel Tsatsouline
Running Time: 1hr 12 minutes
VIDEO **#V110** **$29.95**
DVD **#DV002** **$29.95**

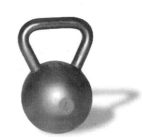

The Sure-Fire Secret to Looking Younger, Leaner and Stronger AN_ Having More Energy to Get a Who_ Lot More Done in the Day

What you'll discover when "Tough" explodes on your monitor:

- The *Snatch*—to eliminate cellulite, firm your butt, and give you the cardio-workout of a lifetime
- The *Swing*— to fry your fat and slenderize hips 'n thighs
- The *Power Breathing Crunch*— to shrink your waist
- The *Deck Squat*— for strength and super-flexiblity
- An incredible exercise to tone your arms and shoulders
- The *Clean-and-Press*— for a magnificent upper body
- The *Overhead Squat*— for explosive leg strength
- The queen of situps— for a flat, flat stomach
- Combination exercises that wallop you with an unbelievable muscular and cardio workout

Spanking graphics, a kick-ass opening, smooth-as-silk camera work, Pavel at his absolute dynamic best, two awesome femme fatales, and a slew of fantastic KB exercises, many of which were not included on the original Russian Kettlebell Challenge video.

At one hour and twenty minutes of rock-solid, cutting-edge information, this video is value-beyond-belief. I challenge any woman worth her salt not to be able to completely transform herself physically with this one tape.

"Kettlebells are without a doubt the most effective strength/endurance conditioning tool out there. I wish I had known about them 15 years ago!"
—*Santiago, Orlando, FL*

"I have practiced Kettlebell training for a year and a half. I now have an anatomy chart back and have gotten MUCH stronger."
—*Samantha Mendelson, Coral Gables, FL*

"I know now that I will never _ into a gym again - who would? absolutely amazing how n individual accomplishment can attained using a kettlebell. Si fantastic. I would recommend anyone at any fitness level, in sport.
—*William Hevener, North Cape May, NJ*

"It is the most effective training I have ever used. I have increased my speed and endurance, with power to boot. It wasn't eve priority, but I lost some bodyfat, w was nice. However, increased ath performance was my main goal, this is where the program r shines."
—*Tyler Hass, Walla Walla, WA*

"In six weeks of kettlebell work, I lo inch off my waist and dropped my hear 6 beats per minute, while staying the weight. I was already working out w started using kettlebells, so I'm not a n There are few ways to lose fat, gain m and improve your cardio fitness all a same time; I've never seen a better one this." —*Steven Justus, Westminster, C_*

Look WAY YOUNGER than Your Age
Have a LEAN, GRACEFUL, Athletic-Looking Body
Feel AMAZING, Feel VIGOROUS, Feel BEAUTIFUL
Have MORE Energy and MORE Strength to
Get MORE Done in Your Day

In Russia, kettlebells have long been revered as the fitness-tool of choice for Olympic athletes, elite special forces and martial artists. The kettlebell's ballistic movement challenges the body to achieve an unparalleled level of physical conditioning and overall strength.

But until now, the astonishing benefits of the Russian kettlebell have been unavailable to all but a few women. Kettlebells have mostly been the sacred preserve of the male professional athlete, the military and other hardcore types. That's about to change, as Russian fitness expert and best selling author PAVEL, delivers the first-ever kettlebell program for women.

It's wild, but women really CAN have it all when they access the magical power of Russian kettlebells. Pavel's uncompromising workouts give *across-the-board, simultaneous, spectacular and immediate results* for all aspects of physical fitness: strength, speed, endurance, fat-burning, you name it. Kettlebells deliver any and everything a woman could want—if she wants to be in the best-shape-ever of her life.

And one handy, super-simple tool—finally available in woman-friendly sizes—does it all. No bulky, expensive machines. No complicated gizmos. No time-devouring trips to the gym.

Into sports? Jump higher. Leap further. Kick faster. Hit harder. Throw harder. Run with newfound speed. Swim with greater power. Endure longer. Wow!

Working hard? Handle stress with ridiculous ease. Blaze thru tasks in half the time. Radiate confidence. Knock 'em dead with your energy and enthusiasm.

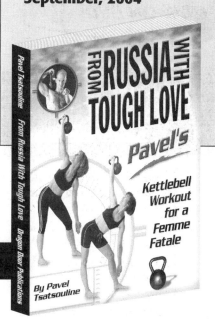

Just some of what *From Russia with Tough Love* reveals:

How the *Snatch* eliminates cellulite, firms your butt, and gives you the cardio-ride of a lifetime

How to get as strong as you want, without bulking up

How the *Swing* melts your fat and blasts your hips 'n thighs

How to supercharge your heart and lungs without aerobics

How to shrink your waist with the *Power Breathing Crunch*
The real secret to great muscle tone

- How the *Deck Squat* makes you super flexible
- An incredible exercise to tone your arms and shoulders
- The *Clean-and-Press*—for a magnificent upper body
- The *Overhead Squat* for explosive leg strength
- Cool combination exercises that deliver an unbelievable muscular and cardiovascular workout in zero time

From Russia with Tough Love
Pavel's Kettlebell Workout for a Femme Fatale
Book By Pavel Tsatsouline
Paperback   184 pages   8.5" x 11"
#B22 $34.95

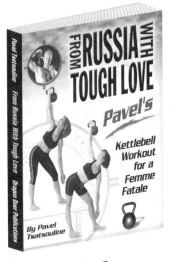

From Russia with Tough Love

Pavel's Kettlebell Workout for a Femme Fatale

Book By Pavel Tsatsouline

Paperback 184 pages 8.5" x 11"

#B22 $34.95

- How to strip away stubborn flab and morph into graceful strength.
- How Russian Kettlebells let you have it all: strength, speed, endurance, and flexibility.
- How Soviet science discovered kettlebell lifting to be one of the best tools for all-around physical development.
- Kettlebells for shoulder and hip flexibility—and as a highly effective tool for strengthening the connective tissues, especially in the back.
- How kettlebells set your fat on fire like no other form of exercise.
- Extra benefits: cheap, indestructible and easy to store.
- How only K-bells deliver strength, explosiveness, flexibility, endurance, and fat loss in one tight package.

What Makes The Kettlebell Workout Unique?

- How KBs strengthen and recruit the deeper, harder-to-work, stabilizing and supporting muscles.
- Gaining greater daily functional strength.
- Why KBs are better at burning off body fat.
- Gives you better muscle definition... stronger tendons and ligaments.

Fast-Track Training Secrets

- How to avoid injuries while gaining strength faster.

- The vital process of synaptic facilitation...how to get more juice of your muscles.
- Succeeding with daily submaximal training...the powerful Russian concept of *continuity of the training process*.
- Your speed lane to fat loss.
- How to get rid of unwanted soreness.
- The delayed training effect...the power of the adaptation lag.
- Intelligent short-term overtraining.

How To Get Very Strong Yet Stay Slender

- Why the mind-muscle link is your real key to strength.
- The structural approach to strength training vs. the functional approach.
- Conscious practice vs. the mindless workout.
- How to rev up recruitment and firing rate to build strength without adding muscle.
- Developing the skill of staying tight for greater safety and performance.
- The real secret to great muscle tone.

Advanced Weight Lifting Secrets

- External and internal resistance training.
- The impracticality of isolation exercises.
- How to optimize full-body tension for your primary muscles.
- How to make heavy metal your best friend.
- How to master the secret of intra-abdominal pressure for greater and safer lifting power...the miraculous effects of Virtual Power Breathing.
- Molding hard obliques... the unexpected benefits of low reps.
- When controlled overtraining or overreaching beats out total recovery training.
- Building up your adaptation reserves for greater gains.
- Little-known secrets that help you grade-out higher on the press.
- How to optimize strength by manipulating the extensor reflex.
- Why locking out your joints is A-Okay.

Get Younger And Healthier With Kettlebells

- Success stories: curing a host of maladies with KBs.
- Rehabilitating hopeless back injuries...from wheelchair to national ranking.
- KBs for better joint health.

Anti-Isolation For Power And Safety

- Why isolation as a key cause of injury in the gym.
- How to take advantage of irradiation for greater strength.
- Maximizing tension with the secret of bracing.
- Using *Starling's law* and the *obtyazhka maneuver* to get stronger in your press.

Think And Be Strong

- The power of thought to make you firmer.
- The Russian sports science concept of skill strength.
- The dating game, iron-style: why's it all about lessons and practice.
- Treating your kettlebell practice as "iron yoga."
- Focusing on the mind, muscle, and breathing connection.

Workouts for the Perfect Female Form

- Unlock the power of your hips with the BOX SQUAT.
- How to improve squatting depth, flexibility, technique, and power.
- Stretch and strengthen your glutes and hamstrings with the GOOD MORNING STRETCH.
- Blast your glutes, hams, inner and outer thighs —and even abs! —with the ONE LEGGED DEADLIFT.
- Strengthen and harden your whole body—and especially your obliques—with the ONE ARM DEADLIFT.
- Firm and shrink your waist, boost your overall strength, and protect your back with the POWER BREATHING CRUNCH.
- Why the conventional crunch is a waste of time and effort...how to avoid neck problems.
- The foolishness of high-rep ab training.
- How to perform Power Breathing for harder abs and a slimmer waist.
- Controlled striking to generate stronger tension.
- Get super flexible and work your hips and thighs even harder with the DECKSQUAT.
- Melt fat and blast your hips and inner thighs with the SWING.
- Get cool and slim with the CLEAN.
- Add power and definition to your hips, thighs, and even abs with the FRONT SQUAT.
- Strengthen and firm your arms and shoulders with the MILITARY PRESS.

- What if I want to work my pec more?— The unique kettlebell floor press.
- The cardio and fat-burning powers of the clean-and-press.
- Strengthen your legs and open your shoulders with the OVERHEAD SQUAT.
- Mold a graceful and athletic body with the TURKISH GETUP.
- Shed cellulite, get a hard butt, and enjoy the cardio workout of a lifetime with the SNATCH.
- How to concoct cool combination exercises that deliver an unbelievable muscular and cardiovascular workout in a very short period.
- The WINDMILL—an unreal drill for a powerful and flexible waist, back, and hip.
- Forge iron wrists and grip and firm up your waist with the BOTTOMS-UP CLEAN-AND-PRESS.
- Get an even harder stomach and tie your upper and lower body into a strong unit with the ROLLING SITUP.
- Cut up your legs and burn calories with the DRAGON WALK—the evil alternative to the lunge.

Freestyle Kettlebell Training

- The tremendous versatility of KBs—fitting your ideal practice schedule.
- Why KB's are NOT for brainless senseless sissies.
- The first commandment of kettlebell training.
- Fragmentation of training volume for more effective strength adaptation.
- The secret power of multiple mini sessions.
- Why fresh and frequent rules.
- Variation cycling for quicker progress.
- When best to practice what.
- Circuit training and the phenomenon of fatigue specificity.
- Two great alternatives to straight sets: Interval training and the ladder, a Russian Special Forces favorite.

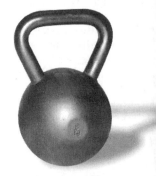

Be as FLEXIBLE as You Want to Be—
FASTER, SAFER and SOONER

I can't say I've read many books on flexibility with the wit and clearheaded wisdom I found in avel Tsatsouline's *Relax Into Stretch*. Tsatsouline delivers the how-and-why of progressive chniques for achieving suppleness, from simple yoga stretching to advance neuromuscular cilitation, without burying the reader in hocus-pocus or scientific jargon. Tsatsouline's *Relax nto Stretch* provides an alternative: straightforward and practical techniques that don't require lifetime to master".

—*Fernando Pages Ruiz, Contributing Editor Yoga Journal*

I tell you truly that *Relax Into Stretch* is superb. Stretching has always been associated with any rious fitness effort and Tsatsouline's approach to this old discipline is fresh and unique and ought provoking. Best of all, this book combines philosophic insight with in-your-face reality s Pavel shares with the reader 'drills' that turn you into what this former Russian Spetznaz istructor calls ' a flexibility mutant'. This book supplies both the road map and the ethodology. Don't ask to borrow my copy."

—*Marty Gallagher, Columnist, WashingtonPost.com*

Pavel Tsatsouline's *Relax Into Stretch: Instant Flexibility Through Mastering Muscle Tension* is superbly illustrated, step-by-step guide to achieve physical flexibility of muscle groups and news. *Relax Into Stretch* is very effective and very highly recommended reading for men and omen of all ages and physical conditions seeking to enhance their mobility and flexibility as part f an overall exercise regimen."

—*Midwest Book Review*

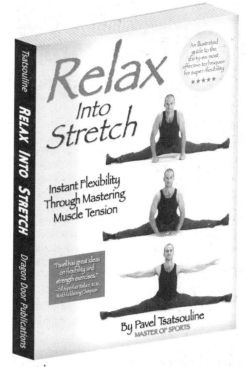

Relax into Stretch
Instant Flexibility Through
Mastering Muscle Tension
Book   By Pavel Tsatsouline
Paperback 150 pages 8.5" x 11"
Over 100 photos and illustrations
#B14 $34.95

- Own an illustrated guide to the thirty-six most effective techniques for super-flexibility
- How the secret of mastering your emotions can add **immediate inches to your stretch**
- How to wait out your tension—the surprising key to greater mobility and a better stretch
- How to fool your reflexes into giving you all the stretch you want
- Why *contract-relax stretching* is 267% more effective than conventional relaxed stretching
- How to breathe your way to greater flexibility
- Using the Russian technique of *Forced Relaxation* as your **ultimate stretching weapon**
- How to stretch when injured—faster, safer ways to heal
- Young, old, male, female—learn what stretches are best for you and what stretches to avoid
- Why excessive flexibility can be detrimental to athletic performance—and how to determine your real flexibility needs
- Plateau-busting strategies for the chronically inflexible.

Relax into Stretch
Instant Flexibility Through Mastering Muscle Tension
By Pavel Tsatsouline
Running time: 37 minutes
Video   #V104   **$29.95**
DVD   #DV006 **$29.95**

Forced Relaxation
Advanced Russian Drills for Extreme Flexibility
By Pavel Tsatsouline
Running time: 21 minutes
Video   #V105   **$24.95**
DVD   #DV007 **$24.95**

Relax Videoor DVD Set:
**Relax into Stretch &
Forced Relaxation**
Video set #VS7   **$49.95**
DVD set #DVS002 **$49.95**

Relax Book and Video Set:
**Relax into Stretch book and Relax into Stretch/
Forced Relaxation videos   #VBS1**
$79.95

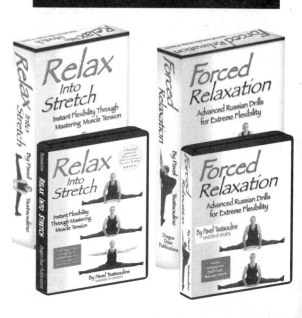

"Injuries Flee the Scene of the Crime, Rehab Miracles Become Norm—Using *Super Joints* Fast Response, Rescue-Your-Own-Body, Super-Relief Program"

"Three days after I initially fractured my elbow I started doing *Super Joints* and within two weeks I had full mobility back in my right arm. I was supposed to attend Occupational Therapy, but when I got there they were so shocked and amazed at my progress that they sent me home. I guess they've never seen someone regain their mobility so fast."—Tonya Ehlebracht, US Army

"*Super Joints* is excellent. It is also saving me a good deal of money. I've had to lay off of heavy squatting and deadlifting because of a back injury. My active release therapist/chiro is amazed at how quickly I am making progress—my alignment doesn't return to crap after an adjustment. I credit the progress mainly to Super Joints." From: chris m., 2003-05-18

"I am 58 and need to keep my joints oiled. I have had very good results with *Super Joints* My knees and elbows don't ache anymore." From: seeahill, 2002-11-07

"I already feel "younger." I'm also noticing an ability to better withstand rolling in Jiu Jitsu class—I don't have to tap quite as often, even in bad positions. Super Joints is a fantastic, fantastic book. I think that everyone should do *Super Joints*." From: Dan McVicker, RKC, 2003-05-18

"As the owner of a sixty-four year old body and as the practitioner of a sedentary job, I have lost some range of motion. The movements in this book have helped me in several ways: 1) Improved the range of rotation of my head. 2) Improved the movement and reduced the pain in the right shoulder injured several years ago. 3) Helped alleviate tension in the neck and traps where I tend to carry stress. 4) Improved my posture helping me look less like a wizened old man."—Comrade Floyd, Amazon.com

"*Super Joints* = Super ROM. Get the book and you'll realize what you've been missing by just stretching. It's more about maintaining the youthful fluidity of the joints which is lost through age and or abuse." From: Larry Dibble, 2002-05-09

Look at all you get to live longer and feel better with *SUPER JOINTS*:

Foreword

Who needs *Super Joints?*...the needs-based survey for super-healthy joint owners...decreasing the odds of injuries...how to develop the right blend of strength and flexibility and improve your survival odds...for better performance...*active flexibility* versus *passive flexibility*...restoring youthful mobility...flexibility development for young athletes...improving posture...kicking-range...improving passive flexibility.

Part One: Joint Health and Mobility

How to keep your one hundred joints running smooth...how *Mobility Drills* can save your joints and prevent or reduce arthritis ...the *theory of limit loads*...Amosov's daily complex of joint mobility exercises...Lying Behind-the-Head Leg Raises...Standing Toe-Touch...Arm Circles... Side bends... Shoulder Blade Reach...Torso Turn...Knee Raises...Pushups...Roman Chair Situps...how to make the Roman chair situp safer...*paradoxical breathing*...squats... the secrets of safer back bending... Amosov's vital tip for creating a surge in your fountain-of-youth calisthenics.

The distinct difference between *joint mobility* and *muscle flexibility* training...Amosov's "three stages of joint health"...appropriate maintenance/prevention strategies for the three stages...how to get started and how to ramp up....the correct tempos for best results—Amosov's way and Pavel's way...when best to perform your mobility drills... shakin' up your proprioceptors—the one-stop care-shop for your inner Tin Man...how to give your nervous system a tune up, your joints a lube-job and your energy a recharge.

From cruise control to full throttle: *The One Thousand Moves Morning Recharge*—Academician Amosov's "bigger bang" calisthenics complex—how to add more cardio and more strengthening to your joint mobility program...adding One Legged Jumps, Stomach Sucks and *The Birch Tree*—how to achieve heaven-on-earth in 25–40 minutes.

Checking yourself...are your joints mobile enough?—F. L. Dolenko's battery of joint mobility tests...four tests for the cervical spine...two for the thoracic and lumbar spine...four for the shoulder girdle...two for the elbows...three for the wrists...three for the hips...and two for the knee joints.

The Drills: Joint Mobility

Illustrated descriptions and special tips:
Three plane neck movements—deceptively simple but great for bad necks...*Shoulder circles*...*Fist exercise*...*Wrist rotations*...*Elbow circles*...how to avoid contracture or age-related shortening...*The Egyptian*—an awesome shoulder loosener popular with Russian martial artists... *Russian Pool*—for super-cranking your shoulders...*Arm circles*—for all the ROM your shoulders need......*Ankle circles*...*Knee circles*...*Squats*...finding the sweet spot...why deep squats are essential and how to avoid injury with correct performance...*Hula hoop*— a favorite of Russian Phys. Ed. Teachers, good for your lower back and hips...*Belly dance*—a must for martial artists...*The Cossack*—a great drill for the hip

joints and your quest for splits...what *never* to do with your knees...*Split switches*—an excellent adjunct to your *Relax into Stretch* split training and simply dandy for your hips...*Spine flexion/extension*...why spine decompression is vital to spine health and mobility...*Spine rotation*...mobility drills for your spine as a top priority for rejuvenation.

Part Two: Strength-Flexibility Plus More Joint Mobility

How to make your body feel better than you can remember...active flexibility for sporting prowess and fewer injuries...*agonists* and *antagonists*...basic active flexibility training...how long to hold an active stretch...how to "Reach the Mark" —using the *ideomotor effect* to successfully extend your stretch... how strength coach Bill Starr develops active and passive flexibility.

How to perform the '*Pink Panther*' technique...taking advantage of the *Ukhtomsky reflex*...how one physical therapist used the Pink Panther to add a couple of feet to her hamstring stretch in one set...the partner hamstring stretch.

Is active isolated stretching any good?—the bottom line on AIS...the demographics of stretching...how and why your age and sex should dictate your choice of stretching exercises...the best techniques for young girls and boys—and what to avoid...a special warning for pregnant women...what adults should do...the elderly...and adolescents.

Stretching to help slumped shoulders...*stretch weakness* and *tight weakness*...how to address the weakness of the overstretched muscles and the tightness of their antagonists...two respected Russian regimens for better posture...understanding the vital difference between a tight and a toned muscle...the *Davis Law*...functional and dysfunctional tension.

The Drills: Strength-Flexibility Plus More Joint Mobility

Illustrated descriptions and special tips:
Windmill—for effectively improving the spine's rotation...*Pink Panther straight-legged situp*—the drill that can add a palm's length to your toe touch in minutes...*Bridge*—awesome for opening up the chest and improving spine extension...some warnings for those with back and wrists problems...how to dramatically improve your bridges with the *Relax into Stretch* hip flexor stretches.

'*Bathtub push*'—opens up the chest, great for posture and a must for a big bench press...how to develop an actively flexible spine with minimal disc loading—three tips from Russian experts...'*Ghost Pulling Knife*'—great for correcting "computer hunch"... *Shoulder dislocate with a bungee cord*—the Olympic weightlifter favorite for mutant shoulder flexibility...*Shoulder blade spread*—a popular stretch among old time strong men...*Side wall reach*...*Pink Panther knee chambers and kicks*—to dramatically improve the height and precision of your kicks...a S.W.A.T. team favorite... a unique stretching technique for high kicks from the Russian army's top hand-to-hand combat instructor...*Pink Panther arabesque*...add more height and power to your kicks with the '*Scissors maneuver*'.

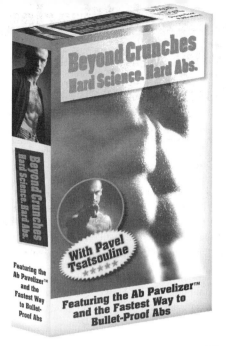

"An Iron Curtain Has Descended Across Your Abs"

Possess a maximum impact training tool for the world's most effective abs, no question. Includes detailed follow-along instructions on how to perform most of the exercises described in the companion book, *Bullet-Proof Abs* Demonstrates advanced techniques for optimizing results with the Ab Pavelizer.

As a former Soviet Union Special Forces conditioning coach, **Pavel Tsatsouline** already knew a thing or two about how to create bullet-stopping abs. Since then, he has combed the world to pry out this select group of primevally powerful ab exercises—guaranteed to yield the fastest, most effective results known to man.

- Fry your abs without the spine-wrecking, neck-jerking stress of traditional crunches.
- No one—but no one—has ever matched Bruce Lee's ripped-beyond-belief abs. What was his favorite exercise? Here it is. Now you can rip your own abs to eye-popping shreds and reclassify yourself as superhuman.
- Russian fighters used this drill, *The Full-Contact Twist*, to increase their striking power and toughen their midsections against blows. An awesome exercise for iron-clad obliques.
- Rapidly download extreme intensity into your situps—with explosive breathing secrets from Asian martial arts.
- Employ a little-known secret from East German research to radically strengthen your situp.
- Do the right thing with "the evil wheel", hit the afterburners and rocket from half-baked to fully-fried abs.
- "Mercy Me!" your obliques will scream when you torture them with the *Saxon Side Bend.*
- How and why to <u>never, never</u> be nice to your abs—and why they'll love you for it.
- A complete workout plan for optimizing your results from the Janda situp and other techniques.

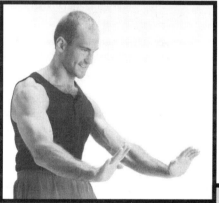

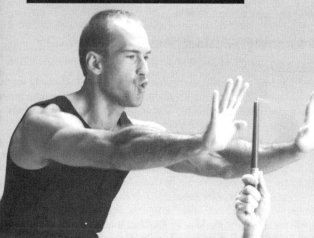

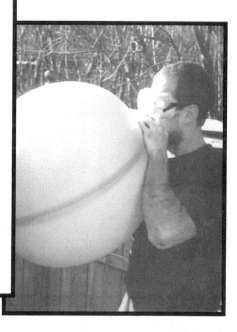

(Right) Pavel's Ab-strengthening breath techniques will give you the power to explode a water bottle—but don't try this trick at home—if the extreme air-pressure whacks back into your lungs, instead of exploding the water bottle—you can end up very dead, which is a bummer for everyone.

(Left) Pavel demonstrates the Power Breathing technique *Bending the Fire* to develop an extra edge in your abs training.

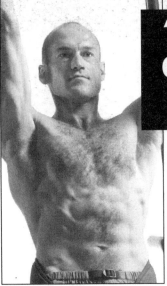

"New Ab Machine Exposes Frauds, Fakes and Cheaters—But Rewards Faithful with the Most Spectacular Abs This Side of Heaven"

The Ab Pavelizer™ II
Item # P12

$139.95
10-25 lb Olympic plate required for correct use.
(You will need to supply your own plate)

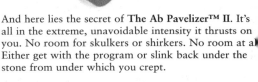
#P12

You know, it's a crying shame to cheat on your abs. Your abs are your very core, your center. Your abs define you, man or woman. So why betray them with neglect and less-than-honest carryings-on? That's bad! And everybody always knows! Rationalize all you want, hide all you want, but weak, flabby abs scream your lack of self-respect to all comers. Why live at all, if you can't hold your head up high and own a flat stomach?

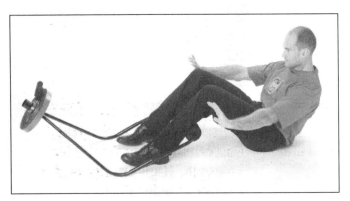

Fortunately, you can now come clean, get honest and give your abs the most challenging, yet rewarding workout of their lives. And believe me, they will love you for ever!

Maybe you've been misled. Maybe you think you have to flog out hundreds of situps to get spectacular abs? Ho! Sorry, **but with abs, repetition is the mother of insanity.** Forget about it! You're just wasting your time! You're just fooling around! No wonder you're still not satisfied!

No, if you <u>really, really</u> want abs-to-die-for then: INTENSITY IS EVERYTHING!

And here lies the secret of **The Ab Pavelizer™ II.** It's all in the extreme, unavoidable intensity it thrusts on you. No room for skulkers or shirkers. No room at all. Either get with the program or slink back under the stone from under which you crept.

You see, The Ab Pavelizer™ II's new sleek-'n-light design guarantees a perfect sit-up by forcing you to do it right. Now, escape or half-measures are impossible. Sit down at the Ab Pavelizer™ II and a divine slab of abs will be served up whether you like it or not. You'll startle yourself in your own mirror!

The secret to the Ab Pavelizer™ II is in the extra-active resistance it provides you. The cunning device literally pushes up against your calves (you'd almost swear it was a cruel, human partner) and forces you to recruit your glutes and hamstrings.

Two wonderful and amazing things happen.

First, it is virtually impossible to do the Janda situp wrong unless you start with a jerk. Second, the exercise becomes MUCH harder than on the Ab Pavelizer™ Classic. And "Much Harder" is Russian for "Quicker Results."

It is astonishingly hard to sit up all the way when the new Ab Pavelizer™ II is loaded with enough weight, 10-35 pounds for most comrades. If you can do three sets of five reps you will already have awesome abs.

A Great Added Benefit: Are you living in an already over-cluttered space? Want to conveniently hide the secret of your abs-success from envious neighbors? The new Ab Pavelizer™ II easily and quickly folds away in a closet or under your bed. Once prying eyes have left you can put it up again in seconds for another handshake with heaven—or hell, depending on your perspective.

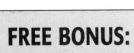
FREE BONUS:

Comes with a four page detailed instruction guide on how to use and get the most out of your Ab Pavelizer™ II. Includes two incredible methods for massively intensifying your ab workout with *Power* and *Paradox Breathing.*

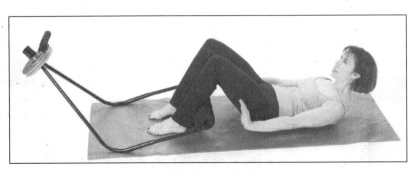

1•800•899•5111 24 HOURS A DAY, OR FAX: (866) 280-7619

When You Unleash the Power of Instinctual Eating

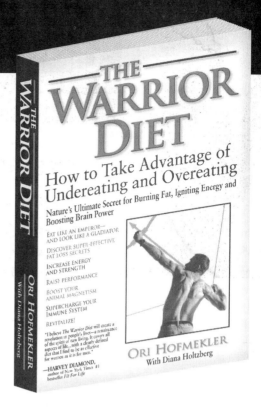

Eat like an emperor—and have a gladiator's body

Are you still confused about what, how and when to eat? Despite the diet books you have read and the programs you have tried, do you still find yourself lacking in energy, carrying excess body fat, and feeling physically run-down? Sexually, do you feel a shadow of your former self?

The problem, according to **Ori Hofmekler**, is that we have lost touch with the natural wisdom of our instinctual drives. We have become the slaves of our own creature comforts—scavenger/victims rather than predator/victors. When to comes to informed-choice, we lack any real sense of personal freedom. The result: ill-advised eating and lifestyle habits that leave us vulnerable to all manner of disease—not to mention obesity and sub-par performance.

The Warrior Diet presents a brilliant and far-reaching solution to our nutritional woes, based on a return to the primal power of our natural instincts.

The first step is to break the chains of our current eating habits. Drawing on a combination of ancient history and modern science, *The Warrior Diet* proves that humans are at their energetic, physical, mental and passionate best when they "undereat" during the day and "overeat" at night. Once you master this essential eating cycle, a new life of explosive vigor and vitality will be yours for the taking.

Unlike so many dietary gurus, Ori Hofmekler has personally followed his diet for over twenty-five years and is a perfect model of *the Warrior Diet's* success—the man is a human dynamo.

Not just a diet, but a whole way of life, *the Warrior Diet* encourages us to seize back the pleasures of being alive—from the most refined to the wild and raw. *The Warrior Diet* is practical, tested, and based in commonsense. Expect results!

The Warrior Diet covers all the bases. As an added bonus, discover delicious Warrior Recipes, a special Warrior Workout, and a line of Warrior Supplements—designed to give you every advantage in the transformation of your life from average to exceptional.

About Ori Hofmekler

Ori **Hofmekler** is a modern Renaissance man whose life has been driven by two passions: art and sports. Hofmekler's formative experience as a young man with the Israeli Special Forces, prompted a lifetime's interest in diets and fitness regimes that would optimize his physical and mental performance.

After the army, Ori attended the Bezalel Academy of Art and the Hebrew University, where he studied art and philosophy and received a degree in Human Sciences.

A world-renowned painter, best known for his controversial political satire, Ori's work has been featured in magazines worldwide, including *Time, Newsweek, Rolling Stone, People, The New Republic* as well as *Penthouse* where he was a monthly columnist for 17 years and Health Editor from 1998–2000. Ori has published two books of political art, *Hofmekler's People,* and *Hofmekler's Gallery.*

As founder, Editor-In-Chief, and Publisher of *Mind & Muscle Power,* a national men's health and fitness magazine, he introduced his Warrior Diet to the public in a monthly column—to immediate acclaim from readers and professionals in the health industry alike.

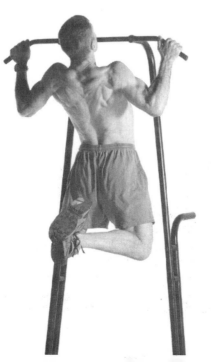

The Warrior Diet

Switch On Your Biological Powerhouse—For Explosive Strength, High Energy and a Leaner, Harder Body
By Ori Hofmekler With Diana Holtzberg

#B23 $24.00
Paperback 420 pages 6" x 9"
#B17 $26.95
Hardcover 420 pages 5 3/8" x 8 3/8"
Over 150 photographs and illustrations

"I believe *The Warrior Diet* will create a revolution in people's lives—a renaissance of the spirit of raw living. It covers all aspects of life... with a clearly defined diet that I find to be as effective for women as it is for men."
—**Harvey Diamond,** author of world bestseller *Fit For Life*

"Rare in books about foods, there is wisdom in the pages of *The Warrior Diet* ...Ori knows the techniques, but he shows you a possibility—a platform for living your life as well...*The Warrior Diet* is a book that talks to all of you—the whole person hidden inside."
—**Udo Erasmus,** author of *Fats That Heal, Fats That Kill*

ORDERING INFORMATION

Customer Service Questions? Please call us between 9:00am–11:00pm EST Monday to Friday at 1-800-899-5111. Local and foreign customers call 513-346-4160 for orders and customer service

100% One-Year Risk-Free Guarantee. If you are not completely satisfied with any product–for any reason, no matter how long after you received it–we'll be happy to give you a prompt exchange, credit, or refund, as you wish. Simply return your purchase to us, and please let us know why you were dissatisfied–it will help us to provide better products and services in the future. *Shipping and handling fees are non-refundable.*

Telephone Orders For faster service you may place your orders by calling Toll Free 24 hours a day, 7 days a week, 365 days per year. When you call, please have your credit card ready.

1·800·899·5111
24 HOURS A DAY
FAX YOUR ORDER (866) 280-7619

Complete and mail with full payment to: Dragon Door Publications, P.O. Box 1097, West Chester, OH 45071

Please print clearly

Sold To: **A**

Name_____

Street_____

City_____

State_____ Zip_____

Day phone*_____
* Important for clarifying questions on orders

Please print clearly

SHIP TO: *(Street address for delivery)* **B**

Name_____

Street_____

City_____

State_____ Zip_____

Email_____

ITEM #	QTY.	ITEM DESCRIPTION	ITEM PRICE	A OR B	TOTAL

HANDLING AND SHIPPING CHARGES · NO COD'S
Total Amount of Order Add:

$00.00 to $24.99 add $5.00	$100.00 to $129.99 add $12.00
$25.00 to $39.99 add $6.00	$130.00 to $169.99 add $14.00
$40.00 to $59.99 add $7.00	$170.00 to $199.99 add $16.00
$60.00 to $99.99 add $10.00	$200.00 to $299.99 add $18.00
	$300.00 and up add $20.00

Canada & Mexico add $8.00. All other countries triple U.S. charges.

Total of Goods	
Shipping Charges	
Rush Charges	
Kettlebell Shipping Charges	
OH residents add 6% sales tax	
MN residents add 6.5% sales tax	
TOTAL ENCLOSED	

METHOD OF PAYMENT ___CHECK ___M.O. ___MASTERCARD ___VISA ___DISCOVER ___AMEX

Account No. *(Please indicate all the numbers on your credit card)*   EXPIRATION DATE

☐☐☐☐ ☐☐☐☐ ☐☐☐☐ ☐☐☐☐   ☐☐/☐☐

Day Phone ( ) _____

SIGNATURE _____ DATE _____

NOTE: We ship best method available for your delivery address. Foreign orders are sent by air. Credit card or International M.O. only. For rush processing of your order, add an additional $10.00 per address. Available on money order & charge card orders only.

Errors and omissions excepted. Prices subject to change without notice.

Warning to foreign customer

The Customs in your country may o
may not tax or otherwise charge yo
an additional fee for goods you
receive. Dragon Door Publications i
charging you only for U.S. handling
and international shipping. Dragon
Door Publications is in no way
responsible for any additional fees
levied by Customs, the carrier or an
other entity.

Do You Have A Friend Who'd Like To Receive A Catalog?

We would be happy to send your friend a free copy. Make sure to print and complete in full:

Name

Address

City   **State**   **Zip**